THE NEW

NOOM DIET COOKBOOK

FOR BEGINNERS

CARLY GOODHART

Copyright

Table of Contents

Introduction

Noom has unquestionably established its part in diets, weight loss programs, and digital health applications. It is clinically proven to help individuals lose weight, and much of its success comes from its behavioural therapy-inspired approach.

The Noom program for weight loss is not a regular diet plan, e.g. there are no off-limit foods or formal eating windows. Noom is more like an all-around lifestyle change that prioritises healthy eating, regular exercise, management of tension, and enhanced sleep hygiene.

Noom's wide-ranging and long-term approach to wellness helps people change their mind and approach weight loss differently. Instead of relying on fast outcomes, Noom teaches people how to change their views on weight and appreciate the value of the physical activity and that healthy nutrition affects a lot more than an amount on a scale.

Nutrition is an essential aspect of Noom's weight loss program as a safe, regular diet is an integral part of long-term weight control. The Noom app is a valuable resource for monitoring progress and offers ongoing guidance from accredited health coaches. Noom uses a colour-coded approach to nutrition: it marks foods as green, yellow or red based on their nutrient density and how much you can consume them.

Noom diet goes past meal plans and calories tracking. It includes a behavioural aspect that could help users dig deeper into why and how to maintain a healthier lifestyle. It is important to remember that this app is not suitable for those dealing with or at risk of eating disorders.

If you want to lose weight, it is essential to consider the caloric density of food, but it is also vital to maintain a balanced relationship with all foods.

At the end, it is up to you whether you want to adopt this diet or move on to some other diet. In this book, you'll find out what the Noom Diet is, what it entails, how it can improve the health of a person. And you will be offered some tasty meals and snacks that are supposed to keep you as healthy as possible while also delivering the results you are looking for.

What is Noom Diet?

If you thrive on mobile apps and virtual interaction, the Noom Diet Plan will work for you. With Noom, it's not only what you're eating, but why you're eating. Noom is about creating self-awareness, responsibility and behaviours that can lead to weight loss and healthy weight management.

You log every meal and snack on the Noom app, plus your normal weight and exercise. Your virtual coach engages with you and inspires you through the messaging feature of the app. You will have a link with your Noom support group mentor and the appointed group members.

Low-calorie foods are the nutritional foundation of the Noom diet, established with the input of registered dietitians. Specifically, Noom promotes foods with a low caloric density, which implies high water quality and lower in calories by volume. Depending on your particular weight-loss target – the weight you intend to achieve at your chosen rate by a specific date – Noom estimates your daily calorie budget.

The Noom organisation has grown from an exercise-and calorie-tracking app to today's strategy that integrates behavioural change science. The staff of Noom includes clinical psychologist Andreas Michaelides. Behaviour modification coaches trained by Noom are chosen for their sympathy and helpfulness, and are not dietitians or nutrition experts.

While Noom has been referred to as a "Millennial Diet," the age spectrum of users is currently reasonably evenly spread between those 18 to 60 years of age and older, with people aged 40 to 59 making up the largest proportion, according to the website.

How does Noom Diet Works?

Download the Noom app and click through a series of questionnaire screens with items such as your weight-loss target, gender, age and starting weight, as well as your desired weight-loss rate. Other screens woven into the mix contain promotional messages, snippets of Noom's ideology, and encouraging study outcomes.

More in-depth demographics discuss your general diet, activity, lifestyle, climate and eating habits, and whether or not you are at risk for a list of diseases, including heart disease, high blood pressure and diabetes. Based on your combined answers, you are told the exact date by which you can meet your target weight.

You're not going to proceed with a detailed meal schedule. Instead, the Noom app responds to the data that you log in to which food and how much you eat. Noom offers three colour-coded food categories to help shape your choices. Foods are grouped by their calorie density and composition of healthy nutrients.

Advantages of Noom Diet

- Certified health coaches
- Psychological approach
- Focus on the long-term
- Emphasis on eating whole foods
- All-in-one support
- Scientifically supported

Disadvantages of Noom Diet

- Expensive
- Language can be somewhat degrading.
- No face-to-face option
- Requires intense commitment

What to Consume?

- Vegetables
- Fruits
- Meats
- Dairy products
- Whole grains
- Healthy fats

What Not to Consume?

- Processed foods
- High fat or greasy foods
- Added sugars
- Oils and condiments

You will find that Noom has a system of colour-coding that separates food into three colors: green, yellow, and red.

Green foods

These foods with the least calorie content per ounces, such as fruit, vegetables and whole grains – are the healthiest options.

Green Food List:

Hearty veggies: Carrots, sweet potatoes, spinach, broccoli, cucumbers

Fruits: Apples, strawberries, oranges, blueberries, apples, bananas, tomatoes

Healthy dairy: Non-fat cheese and non-fat greek yoghurt

Whole grains sides like brown rice & oatmeal, plus alternatives like tofu and almond milk

Yellow foods

Yellow foods, including beans, low-fat cheeses, yogurt, and many low-fat forms of meat, have more calories per ounce. Can make up a moderate proportion of your daily diet.

Yellow Food List:

Lean protein, including tuna, salmon, turkey breast, and grilled chicken

Low-fat milk and yogurt, plus eggs, and other cheeses

Legumes: Black beans and chickpeas

Healthy fats: Avocado and olives

Grains like quinoa and couscous, plus alternatives like whole grain tortillas

Red foods

Red foods contain red meat, juice, nuts, cookies, and pizza and are the most calorie-dense. It should be consumed less often and in smaller portions.

What you should reduce:

Processed meat: Ham, bacon, salami

Oils: Olive oil, coconut oil, and avocado oil

Mayonnaise, ranch, and other heavy condiments

Guilty pleasures: Pizza, hamburgers, fries, chocolate

Sugar, including sources like fruit juice.

Will Noom Diet Help You Lose Weight?

With the Noom Diet plan, you'll probably lose weight. In general, diets that emphasise low-calorie-dense foods have been shown to encourage fullness with less calories and leads to weight loss, and according to Centers for Disease Control and Prevention.

Studies performed by Noom and independent sources support the effectiveness of mobile applications in facilitating and sustaining behavioral improvements in motivated individuals.

Is Noom Diet Safe?

No records have surfaced of significant side effects or threats from pursuing Noom. Noom recommends eating no less than 1,200 calories per day for women and no less than 1,400 calories per day for men for longevity and to ensure that you fulfill your nutritional needs. Noom is built for adults 18 years of age or older.

Although the Noom diet has no common health hazards, those that have had an eating disorder will want to avoid a weight loss program that involves close monitoring of regular eating habits and warns against eating some foods that are still considered healthy.

How Much Should You Exercise On Noom?

Another regular behavior shift that Noom advocates is exercise and simply making you move around. The built-in motion sensor in your smartphone is used by Noom to track your walking by counting your moves. Whenever you're ready, you can increase your phase goal. With the app, you can also track running or multiple other fitness activities.

Is Noom A Heart-Healthy Diet?

Yes, Noom is generally consistent with guidelines from nutritionists and the medical community for a heart-healthy diet. A eating pattern that supports veggies, fruit and whole grains but is low on saturated fats & salt is considered the way to keep cholesterol & blood pressure under control. However, the proposal does not explicitly discuss the reduction of salt. You can monitor your blood pressure readings on the app.

A study published in the Journal of Research in Medical Sciences in May 2016 looked at the impact of a low-calorie diet on cardiovascular risk reduction after recent weight loss. Those on a low-calorie diet decreased their blood levels of total cholesterol and (bad) LDL cholesterol among the 70 participants.

Does Noom Allow For Restrictions And Preferences?

As there are no taboo foods, most individuals may customise Noom to suit their needs.

Recommended supplement?

Noom does not support the use of supplements.

Vegetarian and vegan:

If you're looking for a vegetarian or vegan strategy, Noom is doable. Noom's low calorie density, high-water foods such as vegetables, veggies and whole grains blend well into a vegan or vegetarian style of eating.

Gluten-free:

As part of your regular calorie budget from Noom, you are allowed to choose gluten-free foods.

Low-salt:

If you adopt Noom, low-salt foods are perfect. However, it's up to you to monitor individual low-salt or no-salt products and count your own daily sodium totals.

Kosher:

With Noom, you can keep Kosher—you simply fill in certain foods when your daily meals are logged. However, expressly specified Kosher recipes are not provided by the Noom app.

Halal:

Noom does not provide any halal recipes which are precisely designated.

Healthy Noom Diet recipes are below.

Enjoy!

Sheet Pan Hoisin Chicken

Preparation Time: 12 Minutes

Cook Time: 30 Minutes

Total Time: 40 Minutes

Recipes:

- 2 6-ounce of skinless, boneless chicken breasts
- 1 cup (8 ounces) of small Yukon Gold or red potatoes, halved or quartered
- 2 big carrots sliced into rounds
- 2 cups of broccoli florets
- One red bell pepper cut into chunks
- 1 cup of cauliflower florets
- 2 Tablespoons of olive oil
- salt & black pepper to taste

For the Sauce:

- 1/4 cup of hoisin sauce
- 1/3 cup of minimized sodium soy sauce can substitute with gluten-free tamari or coconut aminos for a paleo-friendly version
- 1 Tablespoon of honey can be substituted with coconut sugar
- 1 Tablespoon of rice wine vinegar
- 2 teaspoons of sesame oil
- 2 cloves of garlic minced
- 1/2 teaspoon of grated or minced ginger
- 1/2 Tablespoon of corn starch

Directions

1. Preheat the oven to 400 °F. For easy clean-up, spray a large nonstick baking pan with oil or use parchment or foil.

2. Put sesame oil, soy sauce, honey, hoisin sauce, ginger, garlic, & cornstarch in a small bowl and set aside.
3. Place the chicken and spread the potatoes over the prepared pan in a single layer. Season the chicken with salt and black pepper on both sides and drizzle with olive oil and sauce.
4. To coat well, toss the potatoes. Cook for 15 minutes and turn on the chicken and potatoes. Drizzle with the remaining vegetables and add the olive oil and sauce.
5. Relating on how thick your chicken pieces are, bake for an additional 15-20 minutes (or until the chicken is completely cooked through).
6. Drizzle with more sauce and sprinkle, if desired, with sesame seeds.

Crispy Sesame Chicken Alongside Sticky Asian Sauce

Preparation Time: 15 Minutes

Cook Time: 15 Minutes

Total Time: 30 Minutes

Recipes:

- 5 tbsp of Vegetable oil
- Two lightly beaten eggs
- Three tbsp of cornflour (cornstarch)
- 10 tbsp of plain (all-purpose) flour
- ½ tsp of salt
- ½ tsp of pepper
- ½ tsp of garlic salt
- 2 tsp of paprika

- Three chicken breast fillets - chopped into bite-size chunks

Sauce:

- 1 tbsp of sesame oil (optional) - you can leave out & just sprinkle with many sesame seeds at the end if you prefer
- Two cloves of garlic - peeled & minced
- One tbsp of Chinese rice vinegar - white wine vinegar will work too
- 2 tbsp of honey
- 2 tbsp of sweet chilli sauce - use more or less depending on the brand & how spicy you like it
- 3 tbsp of ketchup
- 2 tbsp of brown sugar
- 4 tbsp of soy sauce

To Serve:

- Boiled rice
- 2 tbsp of sesame seeds
- Small bunch of spring onions/scallions (chopped)

Directions

1. In a wok or large clean frying pan, heat the oil until very hot.
2. Place the egg in one shallow bowl while the oil heats, and the cornflour in some other shallow bowl.
3. In another shallow bowl, add the pepper, flour, salt, garlic salt, and paprika, and mix.
4. In the cornflour, dredge the chicken, then dip in the egg (make sure that all the chicken is covered in egg wash) & finally dredge it in the seasoned flour. Add to the wok and cook on high heat for 6-7 minutes,

turning until well browned two- or three-times during cooking.

5. You may be required to cook in 2 batches (as long as it's not more than 3 chicken breasts, I find I can do it in one batch). Remove from the pan & place in a kitchen towel-lined bowl.
6. Add all of the sauce recipes to the hot wok, stir & bubble on high heat until the sauce reduces by about a 3rd (should take 2-3 minutes). Add the chicken back in and toss in the sauce to coat. Cook for 1-2 minutes.r
7. Turn the heat off and split it between four bowls. Serve with boiled rice and top with spring onions and sesame seeds.

Herbed Chicken Marsala

Preparation Time: 35 Minutes

Total Time: 35 Minutes

Yields: 4 servings

Recipes:

- Kosher salt
- 4 X (four-ounce) boneless, skinless chicken breast cutlets
- 1/3 cup of whole wheat flour
- Freshly ground black pepper
- 3/4 cup of low-sodium chicken broth
- One and a half tablespoons of extra-virgin olive oil
- Half teaspoon of finely chopped rosemary
- 1/3 cup of sun-dried tomatoes (not packed in oil; not rehydrated), very thinly sliced or finely chopped

- 1/3 cup of sweet marsala wine
- Ten ounces white button or cremini (baby bella) mushrooms, sliced
- One to two tablespoons of roughly chopped flat-leaf parsley
- Two teaspoons of unsalted butter

Directions

1. Firstly, place the chicken cutlets amid two pieces of plastic wrap and then pound using a meat mallet (you can also use a chef's knife) until around 1/3-inch thick. Sprinkle with 1/4 teaspoon of salt and pepper.
2. Now put the flour on a clean medium plate. Heat the oil in a large clean non-stick skillet over medium to high heat. Add in the chicken in the flour, ensure it is thoroughly coat, shake off any surplus. Gently

add the chicken to the skillet and then fry until it is well cooked and turns golden brown, around four minutes for each side. Move to a platter and tent with clean foil to keep warm.

3. Add rosemary, the sun-dried tomatoes, and half a cup of the broth to any remaining drippings in the skillet, and then cook, frequently stirring, for one minute to plump the tomatoes. Now add the mushrooms, half teaspoon of pepper, 1/4 teaspoon of salt, and then cook until the mushrooms get soft, around five minutes.
4. You should add the marsala and then bring it to a boil. Add the 1/4 cup of broth left and the butter and then simmer until the butter is entirely melted, around thirty seconds.

5. Lastly, spoon the mushroom mixture and sauce on top of the chicken, sprinkle with some parsley and then serve to enjoy.

Lemony Yoghurt Pound Cake

Preparation Time: 15 Minutes

Cook Time: 50 Minutes

Total Time: 2 Hours 5 Minutes

Yields: 8 servings

Recipes:

- One and a half cups of white whole wheat flour
- Non-stick baking spray, for coating loaf pan
- Two teaspoons of baking powder
- 3/4 cup of sugar
- 1/4 teaspoon of fine salt
- Half cup of plain low-fat (2%) Greek yoghurt
- Finely grated zest of one lemon
- 1/4 cup of low-fat (1%) milk

- Half teaspoon of pure vanilla extract
- 1/4 cup of extra-virgin olive oil
- One large egg
- Two large egg whites

Directions

1. Oven to 350 degrees Fahrenheit. Gently coat an 8 ½ x 4 ½ -inch loaf pan using a baking spray.
2. Now whisk together baking powder, the flour, and salt in a medium clean container. Add the sugar and lemon zest in a different container and rub the lemon zest into the sugar using your clean fingers. Add milk, the yoghurt, vanilla, olive oil, whole egg, and egg whites, and whisk vigorously until it is evenly blended.

3. You should add the flour mixture into the egg mixture and gently fold until just combined. Move to the readied pan.
4. Proceed to bake until a cake tester in the middle comes out easily, around fifty minutes. Allow pan to cool on a wire rack for five minutes, and unmold.

Lentil Vegetable Soup

Preparation Time: 20 Minutes

Cook Time: 1 Hour 30 Minutes

Total Time: 2 Hours 5 Minutes

Yields: 8 to 10 Servings

Recipes:

- Four cups of chopped yellow onions (three large onions)
- One pound of French green lentils
- Four cups of chopped leeks, white part only (two leeks)
- 1/4 cup of good olive oil, plus extra for drizzling on top
- One tablespoon of minced garlic (three cloves)

- One and a half teaspoons of freshly ground black pepper
- One tablespoon of kosher salt
- One teaspoon of ground cumin
- One tablespoon of minced fresh thyme leaves or one teaspoon dried
- Three cups of medium-diced celery (eight stalks)
- Three quarts chicken stock
- Three cups of medium-diced carrots (4 to 6 carrots)
- 1/4 cup of tomato paste
- Freshly grated Parmesan cheese
- Two tablespoons red wine or red wine vinegar

Directions

1. In a large clean container, cover the lentils with some boiling water and let it sit for fifteen minutes. Drain afterward.

2. In a large clean stockpot on medium heat, sauté the garlic, leeks, and onions with the pepper, olive oil, salt, cumin, and thyme for twenty minutes, until the vegetables are very tender and translucent. Add the carrots and celery and sauté for ten additional minutes. Add tomato paste, lentils, and the chicken stock. Now cover and then bring to a boil.
3. Decrease the heat and then simmer while it is uncovered for one hour, until the lentils are well cooked. Adjust the seasonings if required.
4. Add the red wine and serve while it is hot, drizzled with olive oil and sprinkled with grated Parmesan to enjoy.

Mixed Berries and Banana Smoothie

Preparation Time: 5 Minutes

Total Time: 5 Minutes

Yields: 1 to 2 Servings

Recipes:

- One frozen ripe banana
- One cup of frozen mixed berries
- Half cup of low-fat vanilla yoghurt
- One teaspoon of honey (optional)
- 1/4 cup of orange juice

Directions

Combine all recipes together in a clean blender and puree until it gets smooth.

Slow-Cooker Pork Tacos

Preparation Time: 25 Minutes

Cook Time: 5 Hours 11 Minutes

Total Time: 5 Hour 36 Minutes

Yields: about 8 Servings

Recipes

- Three whole pasilla chiles
- Three whole ancho chiles
- Four cloves of garlic, unpeeled
- Half medium white onion, roughly chopped
- Two to Three chipotles in adobo sauce
- Two tablespoons of honey
- Three tablespoons of extra-virgin olive oil
- One tablespoon of cider vinegar

- Two teaspoons of dried oregano, preferably Mexican
- Kosher salt
- Four pounds boneless pork shoulder (untrimmed), cut into chunks
- 3 3/4 cups of low-sodium chicken broth
- One cinnamon stick
- Freshly ground pepper
- Two bay leaves
- Assorted taco toppings, for garnish
- Corn tortillas, warmed, for serving

Directions

1. Place the pasilla chiles and ancho, and the garlic in a clean container; add two to three tablespoons of water. Now microwave on high heat until it is pliable and soft, two to three minutes. Peel the

garlic; Stem and seed the chiles. Transfer the garlic and chiles to a blender.

2. Add onion, the chipotles, two tablespoons of olive oil, vinegar, honey, the oregano, and one tablespoon of salt to the blender; puree until it gets smooth. Heat one tablespoon of oil left in a large clean skillet over high heat; add the chile sauce and then fry, stirring, until it is thick and begins to fragrant, around eight minutes. Pour in the broth and decrease until just thickened.
3. Season the pork with pepper and salt and move to a large clean slow cooker. Add the cinnamon stick and bay leaves, then gently pour in the sauce. Cover and then cook on high until the meat gets tender, around five hours. (You can as well cook the meat in a Dutch oven, ensure it is covered, for one hour

forty-five minutes at 350 degrees Fahrenheit; Then uncover and cook for thirty additional minutes.)

4. Discard the cinnamon stick and bay leaves. Using two forks, shred the pork; season with pepper and salt. Proceed to serve the shredded pork in the tortillas, along with toppings to enjoy.

Chicken Saltimbocca

Preparation Time: 15 Minutes

Cook Time: 20 Minutes

Total Time: 35 Minutes

Yields: 6 Servings

Recipes:

- Six paper-thin slices of prosciutto
- Salt
- Six (3-ounce) chicken cutlets, pounded to flatten evenly
- Freshly ground black pepper
- Three tablespoons of olive oil
- Two tablespoons of fresh lemon juice

- One (10-ounce) box of frozen chopped spinach, thawed
- One (14-ounce) can of low-salt chicken broth
- 1/4 cup of grated Parmesan

Directions

1. Firstly, place the chicken cutlets flat on the work surface. Carefully sprinkle the chicken with pepper and salt. Lay one slice of prosciutto over each chicken cutlet.
2. You have to squeeze the frozen spinach to discharge the excess water. Season the spinach with pepper and salt. In a small clean container, toss the spinach with one tablespoon of oil to coat evenly.
3. Place in an even, thin layer of spinach over the prosciutto slices. Sprinkle the Parmesan evenly over every of the slices. Starting at the short-tapered end,

roll up every chicken cutlet as for a jellyroll. Protected using a toothpick.

4. In a heavy large skillet over high heat, heat the remaining two tablespoons of oil. Add the chicken and then cook just until it turns golden brown, around two minutes for each side. Add the lemon juice and chicken broth, and the browned bits should be scraped off the bottom of the pan using a clean wooden spoon. Now bring the liquid to a boil. Decrease the heat to medium. Cover and then simmer until the chicken is slightly cooked through, around eight to ten minutes. Move the chicken to a platter.
5. Proceed to simmer the cooking liquid over high heat until it is decreased to around 2/3 cup, approximately five minutes. Season the cooking liquid with pepper and salt, as desired. Get rid of the

toothpicks on the chicken. Drizzle the decreased cooking liquid over the chicken and then serve straight away to enjoy.

Lemon-Garlic Shrimp and Grits

Preparation Time: 15 Minutes

Cook Time: 15 Minutes

Total Time: 30 Minutes

Yields: 4 Servings

Recipes:

- Kosher salt
- 3/4 cup of instant grits
- 1/4 cup of grated Parmesan cheese
- Freshly ground black pepper
- Three tablespoons of unsalted butter
- Two large cloves of garlic, minced
- 1 plus 1/4 pounds of medium shrimp, peeled and deveined, tails intact

- Pinch of cayenne pepper (optional)
- Two tablespoons of roughly chopped fresh parsley
- Juice of half lemon, plus wedges for serving

Directions

1. In a medium clean saucepan over high heat, bring three cups of water to a boil (covered). Uncover and then slowly whisk in the grits, half teaspoon of pepper, and one teaspoon of salt. Decrease the heat to medium to low and cook, occasionally stirring, until it gets thickened, approximately five minutes. Stir in one tablespoon of butter and the Parmesan. Take away from the heat and season with pepper and salt. Cover to preserve the warmth.
2. In the meantime, season the shrimp with pepper and salt. In a large clean skillet over medium to high heat, melt the two tablespoons of butter left. Add

the cayenne, garlic, and shrimp and cook, continually tossing, until the shrimp turns pink, three to four minutes. Take away from the heat and add parsley, two tablespoons of water, and the lemon juice; stir thoroughly to coat the shrimp with the sauce and season with pepper and salt.

3. Split the grits between shallow dishes and then top with the sauce and shrimp. Serve along with lemon wedges to enjoy.

Oil and Vinegar Slaw

Preparation Time: 5 Minutes

Inactive Time: 20 Minutes

Total Time: 25 Minutes

Yields: 6 to 8 servings; leftovers keep 2 days

Recipes:

- Two tablespoons sugar
- 1/4 cup of red wine vinegar
- Two tablespoons peanut or vegetable oil, eyeball it
- One teaspoon of salt
- One sack, 16 ounces, shredded cabbage mix for slaw salads
- Salt
- Pepper

Directions

Mix sugar and vinegar. Add oil. Add cabbage to dressing and season with pepper and salt. Using your fingers, toss to combine. Adjust seasoning if required. Let rest for twenty minutes. Toss again and serve to enjoy.

Blueberry Compote

Preparation Time: 5 Minutes

Cook Time: 18 Minutes

Total Time: 23 Minutes

Yields: 8 Servings

Recipes:

- Three tablespoons of water
- Two cups of frozen blueberries
- Two teaspoons of lemon juice
- 1/4 cup of sugar

Directions

Combine the lemon juice and one cup of the blueberries, water and sugar in a small clean saucepan. Cook over medium heat for around ten minutes. Add the rest of the blueberries and then cook for eight minutes extra, frequently stirring. Serve warm to enjoy.

Shrimp Stir Fry

Preparation Time: 15 Minutes

Total Time: 35 Minutes

Yields: 4 Servings

Recipes:

- One pound of shrimp, peeled and deveined
- Two tablespoons of extra-virgin olive oil
- Kosher salt
- One tablespoon of sesame oil
- Freshly ground black pepper
- Eight ounces of sugar snap peas
- One small head broccoli, cut into small florets
- One red bell pepper, sliced
- One tablespoon of minced ginger
- Three cloves of garlic, minced

- Half cup of low-sodium soy sauce
- Juice of one lime
- One tablespoon of cornstarch
- Pinch red pepper flakes
- Two tablespoons of packed brown sugar

Directions

1. Heat olive oil in a large clean skillet over medium heat. Add shrimp and season with pepper and salt. Cook until it turns pink, five minutes, then take away from the skillet.
2. Take the skillet back to the heat and add sesame oil. Add peas, bell pepper, and broccoli and cook until get soft, seven minutes. Add ginger and garlic and then cook until it begins to fragrant, one minute extra.

3. In a small clean container, whisk together cornstarch, soy sauce, brown sugar, a pinch of red pepper flakes, and lime juice. Add to skillet and then toss to coat evenly. Gently add the shrimp and cook until it is well heated through, two minutes.

Low-Cal Fettuccine Alfredo

Active Time: 25 Minutes

Total Time: 25 Minutes

Yields: 4 Servings

Recipes:

- One clove of garlic, minced
- One tablespoon of unsalted butter
- Two teaspoons of all-purpose flour
- One teaspoon of grated lemon zest
- Kosher salt
- One cup of low-fat (2-percent) milk
- 3/4 cup of grated parmesan cheese, plus more for topping
- Two tablespoons of Neufchâtel or low-fat cream cheese

- Three tablespoons of chopped fresh parsley
- Freshly ground pepper
- Twelve ounces of fresh fettuccine

Directions

1. In a skillet over medium heat, melt the butter. Add the lemon zest and garlic and cook until the garlic is just soft, around one minute. Add in the flour and cook, stirring using a clean wooden spoon, for one minute. Whisk in the 3/4 teaspoon of salt and milk and cook, continually whisking, until slightly thickened, approximately three minutes. Add the parmesan cheese and Neufchâtel; whisk until it is melted, around one minute. Stir in the chopped parsley afterward.
2. In the meantime, bring a large clean pot of salted water to a boil. Add the fettuccine and cook until al

dente (tender), two to three minutes. Reserve one cup of the cooking water, then drain the pasta and return to the pot. Add the sauce and half cup of the reserved cooking water to the pasta and toss gently to combine, adding extra cooking water as required to loosen. Season with salt. Split between dishes and top with pepper and Parmesan.

Marinated Chicken Breasts

Preparation Time: 5 Minutes

Cook Time: 10 Minutes

Total Time: 8 Hours 15 Minutes

Yields: 4 Servings

Recipes:

- two to three teaspoons of dried herbs, like thyme, oregano, rosemary, or crumbled bay leaf
- One to two tablespoons of vinegar, like cider, balsamic, or red wine
- one to two teaspoons of garlic or onion powder, optional
- One to two tablespoons of mustard, whole grain, or Dijon

- Kosher salt
- 1/4 cup of extra-virgin olive oil
- Four boneless, skinless chicken breasts, each about six ounces
- Freshly ground black pepper

Directions

1. Put the herbs, vinegar, powders if using, mustard, and oil in a large clean re-sealable plastic bag. Close the bag and shake to combine all the recipes. Open the bag, place in the chicken breast in the bag. Close and then shake the bag to evenly coat. Freeze for about two weeks.
2. Thaw in the refrigerator overnight, under cold, running water, or in the microwave at thirty percent power for one minute at a time.

3. Proceed to heat a grill pan or grill. As soon as the grill is hot, carefully place the chicken on the grill pan or grill and then cook for approximately four minutes for each side, or until it is well cooked. You can as well bake the thawed chicken in 375 degrees Fahrenheit oven for about fifteen minutes, or until it is well cooked.

Herb-Marinated Pork Tenderloins

Preparation Time: 10 Minutes

Inactive Time: 3 Hours 10 Minutes

Cook Time: 15 Minutes

Total Time: 3 Hours 35 Minutes

Yields: 6 Servings

Recipes:

- 3/4 cup of freshly squeezed lemon juice (4 to 6 lemons)
- One lemon, zest grated
- Two tablespoons of minced garlic (6 cloves)
- Good olive oil
- One tablespoon of chopped fresh thyme leaves

- One and a half tablespoons of minced fresh rosemary leaves
- Kosher salt
- Two teaspoons of Dijon mustard
- Freshly ground black pepper
- Three pork tenderloins (about one pound each)

Directions

1. Combine a half cup of olive oil, lemon zest, lemon juice, garlic, rosemary, thyme, two teaspoons salt, and mustard in a sturdy one-gallon resealable clean plastic bag. Add the pork tenderloins and turn to coat with the marinade. Ensure to squeeze out the air and then seal the bag. Marinate the pork in the refrigerator for at least three hours but if possible overnight.
2. Oven to 400 degrees Fahrenheit.

3. Take out the tenderloins from the marinade and get rid of the marinade but leave the herbs that stick to the meat. Now sprinkle the tenderloins generously with pepper and salt. In a large oven-proof sauté pan over medium to high heat, heat three tablespoons of olive oil. Sear the pork tenderloins on every side until it turns golden brown.
4. Place the sauté pan in the oven and then roast the tenderloins for ten to fifteen minutes or until the meat indicates 137 degrees Fahrenheit at the thickest part. Move the tenderloins to a platter and then cover tightly using clean aluminum foil. Let it rest for ten minutes. Carve in half-inch-thick diagonal slices. The thickest part of the tenderloin will be slightly pink, while the thinnest part will be well done.

5. Season with pepper and salt and serve warm to enjoy, or at room temperature.

Roman-Style Chicken

Preparation Time: 20 Minutes

Cook Time: 40 Minutes

Total Time: 1 Hour

Yields: 6 Servings

Recipes:

- Two skinless chicken thighs, with bones
- Four skinless chicken breast halves, with ribs
- Half teaspoon freshly ground black pepper, plus one teaspoon
- Half teaspoon salt, plus one teaspoon
- One red bell pepper, sliced
- 1/4 cup of olive oil
- Three ounces prosciutto, chopped

- One yellow bell pepper, sliced
- Two cloves of garlic, chopped
- Half cup white wine
- One (15-ounce) can of diced tomatoes
- One tablespoon of fresh thyme leaves
- Two tablespoons of capers
- One teaspoon of fresh oregano leaves
- 1/4 cup of chopped fresh flat-leaf parsley leaves|

Directions

1. Firstly, season the chicken with half a teaspoon of pepper and salt. Heat the olive oil in a large clean skillet over medium heat. As soon as the oil is hot, cook the chicken until it turns brown on all sides. Take the pan off the heat and put it aside.
2. Using the same pan over medium heat, add prosciutto and the peppers and cook until the

prosciutto is crisp and the peppers get browned, around five minutes. Add the garlic and then cook for one minute extra. Add wine, herbs, and the tomatoes. Carefully scrape the browned bits off the bottom of the pan with a wooden spoon. Take the chicken back to the pan, add the stock, and bring to a boil. Decrease the heat and then simmer, covered, until the chicken is well cooked, around twenty to thirty minutes.

3. To serve instantly: add the parsley and the capers. Stir to combine evenly and before serving.
4. If preparing ahead of time: move the sauce and the chicken to a clean container and refrigerate. The next day, heat the chicken again to a simmer over medium heat. Stir in the parsley and capers and serve to enjoy.

Salmon Baked in Foil

Preparation Time: 15 Minutes

Cook Time: 25 Minutes

Total Time: 40 Minutes

Yields: 4 Servings

Recipes:

- Two teaspoons plus two tablespoons of olive oil
- Four (5 ounces each) salmon fillets
- Salt
- Three tomatoes, chopped, or one (14-ounce) can chopped tomatoes, drained
- Freshly ground black pepper
- Two chopped shallots
- One teaspoon dried thyme

- Two tablespoons fresh lemon juice
- One teaspoon dried oregano

Directions

1. Oven to 400 degrees Fahrenheit.
2. Now sprinkle the salmon with pepper, two teaspoons of olive oil, and salt. Stir the shallots, tomatoes, lemon juice, oregano, thyme, two tablespoons of oil, pepper, and salt in a medium clean container to blend.
3. Put a salmon fillet, the oiled side facing down, over a clean sheet of foil. Carefully wrap the ends of the foil to make a spiral shape. Slowly spoon the tomato mixture over the salmon fillet. Gently fold the foil's sides over the tomato mixture and fish, covering; seal the packets. Place the foil packet on a large clean baking sheet. Please do it again until all of the

salmon fillets have been wrapped in different foil and placed on the prepared baking sheet.

4. Proceed to bake until the salmon is slightly cooked, around twenty-five minutes. Move the foil packets to plates using a large clean metal spatula and serve to enjoy.

Roasted Brussel Sprouts

Calories: 184kcal

Preparation Time: 6 Minutes

Cook Time: 22 Minutes

Total Time: 25 Minutes

Yields: 4 Servings

Recipes:

- 1 1/2 lbs of Brussel sprouts (See Note 1)
- 3 tbsp of olive oil separated
- 3/4 tsp of salt
- 1/2 tsp of ground black pepper
- 2 tablespoons of balsamic vinegar
- 2 tsp of honey

Directions

1. Preheat the oven to 425 degreesF.
2. Line up an aluminum foil baking sheet or use a silicone baking mat from Silpat.
3. Trim off the dry outer leaves, cut off the bottom, and lengthwise slice the sprouts.
4. Toss the sprouts with kosher salt & freshly cracked black pepper, and 2 tablespoons of olive oil, in a large clean bowl and coat them thoroughly.
5. Move the Brussel sprouts to the baking sheet but also roast for about 20 minutes, until tender and caramelized.
6. Put the sprouts back in the bowl. Add the remaining tablespoon of olive oil, honey, and balsamic vinegar, and toss to coat evenly. If necessary, taste and season with kosher salt and serve.

One Pan Chicken And Veggies

Recipes:

- Two boneless and skinless chicken breasts
- 1 big sweet potato, diced
- 1 head of broccoli or a large bag of broccoli florets
- 4 cloves of garlic, minced
- 2 tablespoons of fresh rosemary
- 1 tablespoon of paprika
- Salt and pepper to taste
- 2 tablespoons of olive oil

Directions

1. Use a clean aluminum foil to line a baking sheet. Layout all the sweet potato, broccoli, as well as chicken breasts.

2. Spread the garlic, rosemary, paprika, salt, and pepper throughout the pan. Drizzle the olive oil with it.
3. Bake for up till 35 to 40 mins at 400 ° F(or until the chicken's internal temperature reaches 165 ° F & the juices run clear).
4. Serve and have dinner ready! Just toss the aluminum foil carefully for an easy clean-up, and you are good to just go.
5. Enjoy! Enjoy!

Skillet Black Bean Vegetarian Enchiladas Verde

Calories: 403kcal

Total Time: 40 Minutes

Yields: 5 Servings

Recipes:

- Two & a half Tbs of divided Coconut Oil
- 10 (285g) 6" of Corn Tortillas cut into 1" strips - not a mixture of corn & wheat
- 1 cup (112g) of White or Purple Onion medium dice
- 1/2 cup (70g) of Poblano Pepper diced medium, about one small / can sub green bell pepper here
- 1 1/3 cup (160g) of Corn Niblets fresh off the cob or frozen
- 2 tsp of Cumin ground
- 1 tsp of Chili Powder

- 1 tsp of Fine Sea Salt
- 2 cups (235g) of Zucchini medium dice, about 1 medium zucchini
- 15 oz (425g) of Black Beans one can rinsed and drained
- 2 C (500g) of Roasted Tomatillo Salsa Verde, I use homemade
- 1/4 C (60g) of Water
- 1 1/2 C (165g) of Pepper Jack or shredded Monterey Jack Cheese
- Handful Black Olives sliced (optional)

Serve With (optional):

- More tortilla strips, sour cream, limes, avocado, fresh jalapeños, cilantro, sliced tomatoes, salsa.

Directions

1. Add 1 Tbs. of coconut oil to a 10-inch skillet. Heat until it shimmers, over medium-high heat. By tossing and turning the strips, add 1/2 of the tortilla strips until they are all coated with oil. Fry with no flipping or stirring for 3-4 minutes, then starts giving them a toss.
2. Fry for almost ten minutes or until the tortilla strips are a bit charred and golden (as they tend to cool, they will become crisper).
3. To catch any excess grease, remove it from the pan and place it on a paper towel or brown paper. Use a pinch of sea salt to sprinkle. Repeat with the remaining strips of corn tortilla and one tablespoon of coconut oil. Allow to cool and set aside.
4. To the same pan set on a medium-high heat, add the remaining 1/2 Tbs of coconut oil - heat until

shimming. Add the poblano (or green bell pepper) and onions and allow them to sear and become a bit charred. For about four minutes, stirring only occasionally.

5. Add the corn, stir, and allow the veggies to continue charring for another four minutes by just stirring a few times.
6. Add the cumin, chili powder & sea salt to the skillet. Stir to coat all the veggies for about a minute. Add the zucchini, beans, water, and salsa verde. So gently stir & turn the ingredients so that they are incorporated, and nothing falls overboard! The pan will be full.
7. Set aside a cup of tortilla strips and add the remainder to the skillet; add the tortilla strips gently to the rest of the ingredients.

8. Just bring it to a simmer. Put a lid on the skillet and turn the heat to low or medium-low. If or until bubbly, cook for three minutes with the lid on to warm.
9. Sprinkle the cheese well over the top &, if used, slice the black olives. For an additional 2 minutes or more to melt the cheese, put the lid on again. Remove from the heat and immediately serve. Garnish with the tortilla strips remaining and all the toppings you cherish.
10. Store the leftovers in a container for up to three days in the refrigerator or for up to two weeks in the freezer. Thaw for a minimum of eight hours or overnight in the refrigerator. Reheat gently, encased in a 350F (180C) oven.

Cucumber Greek Salad Recipe

Preparation Time: 12 Minutes

Total Time: 10 Minutes

Yields: 8 Servings

Calories: 103kcal

Recipes:

- Two cucumbers peeled & chopped into 1/4 slices
- 4-6 of chopped Roma tomatoes
- Half of red onion, sliced
- 1/4 cup of olive oil
- 1 1/2 Tablespoons of lemon juice
- 2 teaspoons of dried oregano
- 1/2 cup of crumbled feta cheese
- Salt & pepper to taste
- Black olives pitted & sliced (to taste)

Directions

1. Combine the tomatoes, cucumbers, & onions in a large clean bowl.
2. Mix the olive oil, lemon juice, & dried oregano in a smaller bowl. Pour the vegetables over and combine them well. Season the salad with pepper & salt.
3. Sprinkle well the feta cheese on top of the salad with the olives and mix. If necessary, taste and adjust the spices. Until ready to eat, refrigerate. Enjoy! Enjoy!

Sweet Potato Turkey Sliders

Recipes:

- One medium (2- inches diameter, 5- inches long, raw) Sweet Potato (Cooked and Without Salt, Baked in Skin)
- 1/4 serving (serving = 1 tbsp) of Spectrum Organic Virgin Coconut Oil
- 1 cup of Baby Spinach
- 1 serving (serving = 1/4 tsp.) of Mrs. Dash Garlic & Herb Seasoning Blend
- 1 serving (serving = 3 oz) of Trader Joe's Boneless & Skinless Turkey Breast Cutlets

Directions

1. At 375F, Preheat Oven
2. Slice a large sweet potato gently into half-inch discs (and thick in width).

3. Place on the greased sheet of cookies & season (I sprinkled some Mrs. Dash Table Blend on mine)

4. Bake well for 30 minutes before removing it from the oven, flip and bake for 10 more minutes.
5. 3/4 lb grill. Until cooked through, Boneless Turkey Breast (I seasoned mine with Mrs. Dash Garlic & Herb Blend)
6. Cooked turkey sandwich between 2 'buns' of sweet potato with steamed spinach
7. Serve to ENJOY!

Cauliflower Hash Browns

Recipes:

- One large head cauliflower
- ½ cup of parmesan cheese (55 g)
- ⅓ cup of fresh chives (15 g), thinly sliced
- 3 cloves of garlic, minced
- 2 tablespoons of olive oil
- 1 teaspoon of dried basil
- 2 big eggs
- 1 teaspoon of salt, divided
- ½ teaspoon of black pepper
- Dipping sauce (as desired)

Directions

1. Preheat the oven to about 400 °F.
2. Grate the cauliflower with a coarse grater until the entire head has started to crumble down to the small bit.
3. Transfer the bits of cauliflower to a bowl and sprinkle the salt over half a teaspoon. To incorporate the salt, mix the cauliflower and leave to sit for 20 minutes to extract moisture.
4. Transfer the soaked cauliflower to another large towel-lined bowl. Wrap and squeeze the towel shut, so all the excess liquid is strained.
5. Return the cauliflower to the first bowl and add the cheese, chives, garlic, olive oil, basil, black pepper, eggs, and the remaining half a teaspoon of salt to the mixture.

6. Turnover a large roasting tray and parchment paper line - this helps prevent hash browns from burning on the bottom. Divide the mixture of cauliflower into 6 even pieces, place on the tray as well as shape into hash browns.
7. Bake until golden brown, for 35-40 minutes.
8. Let the hash browns cool until they have set for about 15 minutes.
9. Serve the desired dipping sauce with it.

Vegan Creamy Mushroom Ramen

Preparation Time: 3 Minutes

Cook Time: 12 Minutes

Total Time: 15 Minutes

Yields: 1 Servings

Recipes:

- 1/2 Tbsp of cooking oil
- 4 oz. of baby Bella mushrooms
- 1.5 cups of vegetable broth
- 1 handful of fresh spinach
- 1 package of ramen noodles (discard seasoning)
- 1/2 cup of coconut milk (canned)

Optional Garnishes:

- One green onion, sliced
- 1 Tbsp of chili garlic sriracha or sauce

Directions

1. Gently Slice the mushrooms. Add them to the cooking oil in a small saucepot & sauté over medium heat until the mushrooms are soft, dark & all the moisture has evaporated from the bottom of the pot.
2. Turn the heat to medium-high, add the vegetable broth, and bring the broth to a boil. Upon boiling, add the ramen noodles to the broth (but without sauce packet). In the boiling broth, cook the noodles for about 3 minutes, or till tender.
3. Turn off the heat & a handful of fresh spinach to the heap, and stir until the spinach wilts (about 30 seconds). Into the pot, pour the coconut milk & stir to combine.
4. Serve as-is, or with garnishes like green onion or chili garlic sauce, the Vegan Creamy Coconut Ramen.

Easy Vegan Mac And Cheese

Recipes:

- One box of Whole Wheat or Gluten-free Pasta use any pasta of choice
- Two big Yukon Gold Potatoes
- Three Medium Carrots
- Two cups of Broccoli Florets
- Two cloves of Minced Garlic
- A quarter Cup of Nutritional Yeast
- One Tsp of Apple Cider Vinegar
- Two Tbsps. of Freshly-Squeezed Lemon Juice
- 1 Tsp of Dijon Mustard
- A half Tsp of Paprika
- ⅛ Tsp of Turmeric Powder
- A half tsp of Kosher Salt
- A quarter tsp of Ground Pepper

Directions

1. To remove any dirt, wash and thoroughly scrub the potatoes and carrots. Peel off the skin of the potatoes & carrots using a potato peeler and cut into big bite-sized chunks.
2. In a large pot, add chopped potatoes and carrots, then pour over enough water to cover 1 inch. Season with a friendly pinch of salt and bring water, over medium-high heat, to a boil.
3. Simmer for 15 minutes or until a paring knife easily pierces the potatoes and carrots underneath cold running water. With a clean paper towel, pat out the surplus moisture.
4. Meanwhile, under another pot filled with about 1 cup of water, add a steamer basket (or make use of the same pot where the veggies are boiling if the steamer does not touch the water). Steam the

broccoli for 3-4 mins, or just until the fork-tender is tender.

5. Remove from the heat once the veggies are done and place in a colander to drain, reserving approximately 1 cup of water from the veggies. Allow slightly to cool the veggies. Then according to package directions, cook the pasta.
6. Combine the apple cider vinegar, garlic, lemon juice, mustard, paprika, turmeric, & salt whisk in a small clean mixing bowl until well combined and set aside.
7. Next, place in a blender the boiled potatoes, carrots, dietary yeast, and 1/2 cup of the reserved liquid.
8. Pour in the mixture of prepared garlic and vinegar and mix until smooth and creamy, for about 2-3 minutes. To reach your desired consistency, add more liquid if needed.

9. In a large serving bowl, add the cooked pasta together with the steamed broccoli, then pour the sauce on top.
10. Mix well with a clean wooden spoon until the pasta is evenly coated in the super delicious creamy sauce! Serve it hot and enjoy it!

Vegan Spinach Avocado Pasta Recipe

Recipes:

- 10 ounces of whole-wheat spaghetti
- One ripe avocado peeled & seeded
- One cup of fresh spinach leaves
- A half teaspoon of minced garlic
- One tablespoon of olive oil
- One tablespoon of lemon juice
- Salt & pepper to taste
- One and a half cups of cherry tomatoes halved
- Two tablespoons of toasted pine nuts
- Two tablespoons of chopped fresh parsley

Directions

1. Cook the pasta according to package procedures in salted water. Set aside a quarter cup of the cooking water.

2. Make the sause whilst the pasta is undergoing cooking. In a food processor, put the spinach, avocado, garlic, olive oil, lemon juice, a half teaspoon of salt & a quarter teaspoon of pepper.
3. Blend and add 1 tablespoon of cooking water at a time until the sauce is smooth and has the desired consistency. When necessary, taste and add further salt & pepper.
4. With the sauce, toss the pasta. Serve immediately with cherry tomatoes, pine nuts, as well as parsley.

Creamy Zucchini Sauce

Preparation Time: 10 Minutes

Cook Time: 20 Minutes

Total Time: 30 Minutes

Recipes:

For Zucchini:

- 2 lbs. of zucchini cubed
- 3 tbsp. of olive oil
- 1 tbsp. of paprika
- pepper & salt to taste

For the Sauce:

- 1 cup of sour cream
- 2 garlic of cloves minced
- 1 tbsp. of tomato paste
- 2 tbsp. of chopped dill

- 2 tbsp. of chopped basil
- Salt to taste

Directions

1. Gently preheat the oven to 400° F.
2. Use a clean large nonstick baking tray to mix the zucchini with oil, paprika, salt, and pepper. Bake for 20 minutes or so, until tender but also lightly browned.
3. Meanwhile, in a medium skillet, place all the sauce ingredients, stir and bring to a simmer. Switch the heat off.
4. For the cream sauce, add the baked zucchini and mix everything well. If desired, garnish it with chopped herbs.

Cheesy Chimichurri Broccoli

Total Time: 20 Minutes

Yields: 6 Servings

Recipes:

- Olive oil
- A half-cup of avocado mayo
- Haven's Kitchen Herby Chimichurri
- One & a half cups of grated cheddar, divided
- Two heads of broccoli (Strictly florets)

Directions

1. Preheat the oven to 400°F. In salted water, boil or steam the broccoli until tender (about 4-5 mins). Use olive oil to grease a 2-quart baking dish.
2. Combine the mayonnaise, 1⁄4 pocket of Chimichurri, and half of the cheddar in a large bowl.

3. Add the cooked broccoli to the creamy sauce by scooping it directly from the clean pot to the bowl. Gently toss to coat.
4. Move the coated broccoli to the clean baking dish. Sprinkle on the remaining cheddar.
5. Bake the broccoli until the edges are golden brown and bubbly for about 15 minutes. For a super crispy top, broil for another 3-5 minutes.

Vegan Jambalaya

Recipes:

- One diced onion
- Two stalks of celery, chopped
- Four cloves of garlic, minced
- A half diced green pepper
- A half diced red pepper
- One can (400 grams / 14 oz) of crushed tomatoes
- 4 cups (1 litre) of vegetable stock
- 1 teaspoon of dried oregano
- 1 teaspoon of dried basil
- 1 teaspoon of dried thyme
- 1 teaspoon of sweet paprika
- ½ teaspoon of smoky paprika
- ½ teaspoon of dried cayenne pepper
- Two bay leaves

- Two tablespoons of Tabasco sauce (adjust to taste)
- Two tablespoons of soy sauce
- Pepper for taste
- 2 cups (400 grams) of uncooked brown rice
- 3 cups (500 grams) of mixed beans (I used chickpeas, white beans, and kidney beans)
- 1 teaspoon of salt (to taste)
- ¼ cup (7 grams) of fresh chopped parsley
- One chopped green onion (optional)

Directions

1. Over medium-high heat, heat a large pan and add a splash of water or a tablespoon of oil to it. Add the garlic & onion & sauté until soft. Add the celery and peppers and, if necessary, another splash of water, and sauté until the softening begins.

2. Add crushed tomatoes, herbs, vegetable stock, spices, and sauces (with the exception of salt), and rice to the mixture. Bring to a boil & then lessen the heat to a low level and cover the pan. Simmer gently for to 40 mins until the rice is cooked and the fluid is absorbed. At the end of the cooking period, keep an eye on it, and stir from time to time to prevent the rice from trying to stick.
3. Stir in the beans and taste once the rice is tender. If necessary, add salt. For those who like it really spicy, give it a minute to heat the beans, then proceed to serve the jambalaya with fresh chopped parsley & green onion sprinkled on top and more Tabasco sauce on the side.

Farfalle Pasta With Spinach, Caramelized Onions, And Mushrooms

Preparation Time: 20 Minutes

Cook Time: 30 Minutes

Total Time: 50 Minutes

Recipes:

- Plenty Caramelized onions
- 1 tablespoon of olive oil
- 3 large yellow onions, sliced
- 1/4 teaspoon of salt
- 1 tablespoon of balsamic vinegar
- Creamy pasta sauce
- 1 tablespoon of olive oil
- 10 oz of mushrooms, sliced (I made use of button mushrooms)
- 6 oz of spinach

- 1 cup of half-and-half
- 1 cup of shredded Parmesan cheese
- 1/4 teaspoon of salt
- Pasta
- 8 oz of farfalle pasta

For the caramelize onions:

1. On a medium-high heat, heat 1 tablespoon of olive oil in a large skillet. Add the sliced onions & cook it for about 10 minutes, constantly stirring with the spatula, over high heat.
2. It should begin to brown the onions, but without burning.
3. Reduce heat to medium and continue to cook onions for an additional 10 minutes, stirring further, browning onions even more without burning. Put a pinch of salt over the onions at this point.

4. On medium or low heat, continue cooking for 10 more minutes, stirring occasionally to make sure the onions do not stick to the bottom of the pan or burn.
5. In total, you should have 30 minutes of cooked onions.
6. Gently remove the skillet from the heat & pour a small amount of balsamic vinegar over the onions to deglaze the pan.
7. Stir the onions with a spatula, scrape the bottom of the pan and coat the onions with a pinch of the balsamic vinegar you have just added. On a plate, remove the caramelized onions.

For the mushrooms and spinach:

1. On a medium heat, heat one tablespoon of olive oil in the same skillet. Add the sliced fungi. Use a pinch of salt to sprinkle.

2. Cook the mushrooms for approximately 5 minutes, occasionally stirring, until they are soft.
3. Add the fresh spinach to the skillet and stir until the spinach begins to wilt.

For the creamy pasta sauce:

1. Add the mushroom and spinach mixture to half-and-a-half and bring to a quick boil. Decrease immediately to simmer.
2. Add 2/3 of a cup of Parmesan shredded cheese and 1/4 of a teaspoon of salt. Keep stirring until the cheese melts while the sauce simmers.
3. Add the caramelized onions and the pasta sauce back to the skillet.

For the Pasta:

1. Cook pasta in reference to the instructions in the package. Uh, drain.

2. For the creamy sauce, add cooked and drained farfalle pasta. Stir well for a few minutes on low heat to reheat.
3. Add a little amount of half-and-half to thin it out if the sauce is too thick. Add a little amount of shredded Parmesan cheese if it is too thin, and stir it in while the sauce is simmering.
4. Serve with sprinklings of more shredded parmesan cheese.

Garlic Butter Turkey Meatballs Also With Lemon Zucchini Noodles

Preparation Time: 15 Minutes

Cook Time: 15 Minutes

Yields: 4 Servings

Recipes:

- 1/2 lb (220g) of ground turkey meat
- 1/2 lb (220g) of ground pork meat (optional, see recipe notes)
- 1/2 cup of shredded mozzarella
- 4 cloves of garlic, grated with two cloves garlic, minced
- 1 teaspoon of Italian seasoning
- 1/2 teaspoon of red crushed chili pepper flakes (optional)
- One crumbled bouillon cube (optional)

- Salt & fresh cracked black pepper for taste
- One cup of fresh chopped cilantro (or parsley), divided
- 3 tablespoons of butter
- Four medium zucchinis, spiralized
- A half lemon juice
- One tablespoon of hot sauce of your choosing(I made use of Sriracha)

Directions

1. Combine ground turkey with ground pork, cheese, grated garlic, Italian seasoning, red chili pepper flakes, bouillon cube, chopped cilantro, and black pepper in a large bowl. With your hands or fork, mix well and form medium balls. On a plate, arrange the turkey meatballs and set them aside.

2. Melt two tablespoons of butter over a medium-low heat in a large skillet. On all sides, cook the turkey meatballs for 8-10 minutes, until browned and cooked. Baste the meatballs with a mixture of butter and juices while you cook. Remove and set aside on a clean plate.
3. Melt the rest tablespoon of butter in the same clean skillet, then add the lemon juice, hot sauce, minced garlic & red pepper flakes (if you want). Add the zucchini noodles & cook, stirring regularly, for 3 or 4 minutes, until the zucchini is done but still crisp and the juices are slightly reduced. Adjust the salt and pepper seasoning and garnish with more coriander or parsley if you want some.
4. On one side of the skillet, push the zucchini and add the turkey meatballs back into the pan & reheat for a minute or two. Serve immediately with a lemon slice

on the side of the garlic butter turkey meatballs with lemon zucchini noodles. Enjoy! Enjoy!

One Pot Turkey Chili Mac And Cheese

Preparation Time: 10 Minutes

Cook Time: 25 Minutes

Total Time: 35 Minutes

Yields: 8 Servings

Calories: 359kcal

Recipes:

- One lb of ground turkey
- One diced onion finely
- One teaspoon of salt
- Three cups of chicken broth
- Two cans (8 oz each) of tomato sauce
- One can (15 oz) of pinto beans drained & rinsed
- 2 teaspoons of chili powder
- 1 teaspoon of cumin

- 1 teaspoon of garlic powder
- A half teaspoon of cocoa powder
- 3 cups of small shell pasta (dry, do not cook beforehand)
- 2 cups of shredded cheese (I use Colby Jack)

Directions

1. Cook & crumble the ground turkey, onion & salt in a large skillet over medium-high heat until the turkey is no longer pink. Drain any surplus liquid (there will be many from the turkey)
2. Add the tomato sauce, chicken broth, pinto beans, chili powder, cumin, garlic powder, and cocoa powder to the bowl. Stir and bring to a boil.
3. Add in the dry pasta after boiling and bring it to a boil. Decrease the heat to medium-low after boiling

and cover with the lid. Cook for 15-20 or until you have absorbed all the liquid.

4. Take off the lid and add the cheese that has been shredded. Stir so that the cheese is combined and melted. Now it's ready to eat!
5. If desired, it can be served with sour cream, green onions, and additional shredded cheese.

Baked Spinach Provolone Chicken Breasts

Preparation Time: 5 Minutes

Cook Time: 35 Minutes

Total Time: 40 Minutes

Yields: 2 Servings

Recipes:

- Two boneless & skinless Chicken Breasts butterflied
- Two slices of Provolone cheese
- One 5 oz of container of fresh Baby Spinach
- 4 cloves of minced garlic
- A dash of Paprika
- One Tablespoon of Olive Oil

Directions

1. Preheat the oven to 425°C.

2. Add the olive oil and garlic to the large frying pan, and sauté for 1-2 minutes over medium heat.
3. Add the spinach and often stir, about 2-3 minutes, until the spinach is wilted and cooked.
4. Butterfly chicken breasts are sliced down the middle lengthwise, but not all of the way through.
5. Over each chicken breast, put a slice of Provolone cheese.
6. Add the whole spinach on top of the cheese & the garlic.
7. Fold the chicken in half like a sandwich to keep the stuffing inside.
8. Place it on a greased baking tray.
9. Sprinkle the chicken with paprika on top.
10. 30 Minutes of Bake Uncovered.
11. Serve to Enjoy!

Zucchini Pizza Crust

Preparation Time: 15 Minutes

Total Time: 50 Minutes

Yields: 4 – 6 Servings

Recipes:

- 3 medium zucchinis, or about Four cups grated zucchini
- One big egg
- Two cloves of minced garlic
- 1/2 tsp. of dried oregano
- 3 c. of shredded mozzarella, divided
- 1/2 c. of grated Parmesan
- 1/4 c. of cornstarch
- kosher salt
- Ground black pepper (Fresh)
- 1/4 c. of pizza sauce

- 1/4 c. of pepperoni
- A pinch of red pepper flakes, for garnish
- Basil (for garnish)

Directions

1. Preheat the oven to 425 degrees and line a parchment baking sheet. Grate the whole zucchini in a food processor. Squeeze the excess moisture out of the zucchini using a cheesecloth or a dish towel.
2. Mix the zucchini with the egg, garlic, oregano, 1 cup of mozzarella, Parmesan, and cornstarch in a large clean bowl & season with salt & pepper. Stir until combined entirely.
3. To the prepared baking sheet, transfer the dough and pat it into a crust. Bake for 25 minutes until they are golden and dried out.

4. Spread well the pizza sauce all over the crust & top it with the remaining pepperoni and mozzarella. Bake for 10 more minutes until the whole cheese is melted and the crust is crispy. Add red pepper flakes and basil to garnish.

Cauliflower Crust Pizza

Active Time: 35 Min

Total: 1 Hour 50 Min (Includes Cooling Time)

Yield: 2 Servings (1 Pizza)

Recipes:

For Pizza:

- 1 medium of head cauliflower, cut into florets
- 1/4 cup of grated Parmesan
- 1 teaspoon of Italian seasoning
- 1/4 teaspoon of kosher salt
- 1 big egg
- 2 cups of freshly grated mozzarella
- 1/4 cup of Spicy Pizza Sauce, recipe follows
- Freshly basil leaves, for the purpose of garnish

For Salad:

- 4 cups of baby greens
- 2 tablespoons of olive oil
- 1 tablespoon of balsamic vinegar
- Kosher salt & freshly ground black pepper
- Parmesan shavings, for the purpose of topping

Spicy Pizza Sauce:

- 1 to 2 tablespoons of olive oil
- Three cloves of garlic, minced
- One medium onion, finely chopped
- A half-cup of chicken broth
- 3 15-ounce cans of crushed tomatoes
- 1 tablespoon of brown sugar
- 1 teaspoon of red pepper flakes
- Kosher salt & freshly ground black pepper

Directions

1. For pizza: Preheat the oven to a temperature of 425 degrees F. With parchment paper, line a rimmed baking sheet.
2. Pulse the cauliflower florets into a fine snowy powder in a food processor (you should have about 2 1/2 cups). To a microwave-safe bowl, transfer the processed cauliflower and cover until soft, microwave for 4 to 6 minutes. Transfer to and allow to cool on a clean, dry kitchen towel.
3. Wrap the cauliflower in the towel & wring out as much moisture as possible when cool enough to handle, transferring if necessary, to a second towel.
4. Stir the cauliflower, Parmesan, Italian seasoning, salt, egg, and 1 cup of mozzarella together in a large bowl until well combined. Transfer to the baking

sheet that has been prepared and press into a 10-inch round. Bake for 10 to 15 minutes until golden.

5. Take the crust from the oven & top with the remaining 1 cup mozzarella and the Spicy Pizza Sauce. Bake for ten more minutes, until the whole cheese is melted and bubbly. Just before serving, garnish it with fresh basil leaves.
6. For the salad: Meanwhile, in a large clean bowl, add the greens. In a measuring cup, whisk together the balsamic oil, olive oil, salt, and pepper to taste. Pour and toss over the greens. Top with shavings of Parmesan.

Spicy Pizza Sauce:

Yield: One and a half cups

1. Heat a pan until warm, over medium-high heat. Add a tablespoon of olive oil & stir in the garlic and

chopped onions. Cook for 4 to 5 minutes, until the onions are soft. To deglaze the bottom of the pan, whisk in the chicken broth.

2. Cook until you have reduced the liquid by half. To combine, add the crushed tomatoes and stir. To taste and stir, add the brown sugar, red pepper flakes, and salt and pepper. Bring to a simmer, bring it to a low heat and simmer for 30 minutes. Let the sauce cool, then puree it.

Spinach Stuffed Chicken Breast

Preparation Time: 15 Minutes

Cook Time: 30 Minutes

Total Time: 45 Minutes

Recipes:

- Four chicken breasts approximately 2 lbs.
- 4 oz. of fresh baby spinach
- 4 oz. of cream cheese
- 2 oz. of feta cheese crumbles
- 2 oz. of shredded mozzarella cheese
- 2 tbsp. of olive oil

Seasoning ingredients:

- 2 tsp. of paprika
- 1 tsp. of cumin powder
- 1 tsp. of salt

- 1/2 tsp. of chili powder

Directions

1. Mix together all the seasoning ingredients and set them aside.
2. Chop the baby spinach roughly and place it into a mixing bowl. Add the cream cheese, mozzarella, and feta.
3. Massage your hands with the spinach until well combined (it should look like thick paste).
4. Gently cut a pocket into both sides of each chicken breast with the help of a sharp knife.
5. Divide the stuffing of the spinach into four equal parts and spoon it into the pockets of the chicken. Secure the stuffing inside by using toothpicks.
6. Season the chicken well with the spice mix & brush on both sides with olive oil.

7. As regards on how big your chicken breasts are, bake the chicken in a preheated oven at 400oF for 25-30 minutes.

Peppered Beef With Sweet Potato Mash

Yields: 4 Servings

Recipes:

- 1 kg of Buccleuch beef eye fillet (or alternative beef fillet)
- 1 tbsp of freshly ground black pepper
- 1 tbsp of grain mustard
- 1 kg of orange-fleshed sweet potatoes
- 120g of butter
- One small bunch chive, finely chopped

Directions

1. Preheat the furnace to 2000C.

2. Trim the beef fillet and rub the surface with the mustard and freshly ground pepper. Place it overnight on a tray in the fridge.
3. Place the fillet in a baking pan and roast for 10-15 minutes when ready to cook. Just remove it from the oven and keep it warm.
4. Meanwhile, the sweet potatoes are peeled and boiled in plenty of water, drained when soft and ready, and mashed into a fluffy mash along with the butter. Have the chopped chives added and keep it warm
5. Place the fillet back in the oven & cook for an additional 10 minutes if you like medium-rare meat or another 15 minutes for medium to well-done meat.
6. Use a dollop of sweet potato mash to slice the beef fillet and serve.

Sweet Garlic Chicken

Recipes:

- Two Chicken Breasts
- A half tsp of each Salt & Pepper
- Two tbsps. of Olive Oil and more for drizzling
- Three Cloves of Garlic, minced
- 2 tbsps. of Brown Sugar

Directions

1. Gently preheat the oven to 450 F.
2. Place the breasts of the chicken in a baking dish. (Using nonstick foil, I advise. There is a lot of mess leftover once this is cooked. It just makes cleaning easier.) Drizzle with olive oil lightly and sprinkle with salt and pepper on both sides.

3. Heat 2 tablespoons olive oil over medium heat in a saucepan. In heated oil, add minced garlic. Cook for around 2 minutes till it becomes softened.
4. Turn the heat off, then add the brown sugar. Until combined, stirring. Spread the mixture of brown sugar evenly over each part of the side facing up.
5. Bake the chicken for 15-20 minutes when the oven is warm. Remove and serve as well.
6. I would use 1 tbsp of olive oil and 1 tbsp of brown sugar per breast if I were to feed more than two people, and garlic to taste. Enjoy! Enjoy!

Spinach Stuffed Chicken Breasts

Preparation Time: 10 minutes

Total Time: 25 minutes

Cook Time: 15 minutes

Yields: 6 Servings

Calories: 434kcal

Recipes:

- Three chicken breasts
- 8 oz of chopped frozen spinach cooked according to package procedures & squeezed dry.
- 3 oz of feta crumbled (about a half cup)
- 4 oz of cream cheese
- 1 clove of garlic diced
- 1/4 teaspoon of salt divided
- 1/8 teaspoon of pepper

- 1 tablespoon of olive oil

Directions

1. Gently preheat the oven to 450 degrees F.
2. In a medium-sized bowl, mix the chopped frozen spinach, feta, cream cheese, garlic, and half of the salt.
3. Into each chicken breast, cut a pocket. one at a time, place the whole chicken flat on a clean cutting board, and press a large spatula (or something else that can't be stabbed, i.e., DO NOT USE MAKE USE OF YOUR BARE HAND) flat on top of the breast if you're unsure how to cut a pocket into the chicken without cutting a pocket into your hand as well. Ensure that you are pressing the spatula down hard enough to hold the chicken in place.

4. In fact, you may need to dig the edge of the spatula into the meat just a little bit to achieve this. Insert the knife into the part of the thickest part of the chicken 2/3 of the way, and slice down to the thinnest part, stopping before cutting through; you don't want a flap for a pocket.
5. Separate the mixture of spinach and cheese into three parts, then roll it into thick logs. Stuff each log into the pocket of the chicken breasts you made. Season with the remaining pepper and salt.
6. In an oven proof pan set over medium-high heat, heat the olive oil and then add the stuffed chicken, "top" side down. 5 minutes to cook, then flip the chicken over.
7. Put the pan in the oven & let it cook for 10 minutes. Cook for 2 to 5 minutes longer if your chicken

breasts are extraordinarily thick, or until the juices are clear when you poke the chicken with a fork.

Parmesan Crusted Potatoes

Preparation Time: 10 Minutes

Cook Time: 45 Minutes

Total Time: 55 Minutes

Recipes:

- 5 medium red potatoes, peeled
- A half-cup of grated Parmesan cheese
- 1 tsp of paprika
- 1 tsp of garlic powder
- 3 tbsp of olive oil
- salt for taste
- chopped fresh parsley to garnish it

Directions

1. Cut the potatoes into pieces that are 1/2 inch thick (refer to the photo above).

2. Place the potatoes and add the rest of the ingredients, excluding parsley, in a medium mixing bowl. Mix well everything.
3. Set the potatoes in a single layering on a clean baking sheet. To stop the potatoes from sticking to the sheet, I recommend using parchment paper or a silicone mat.
4. Bake at 450F for about 25-30 minutes in a preheated oven. Take them out of the oven, flip over each piece, and bake for 10-15 more minutes.
5. With some chopped parsley or grated Parmesan, garnish the potatoes.

Spaghetti Squash Sausage Lasagna Boats

Course: Dinner

Yield: 6 Servings

Recipes:

- 3 small to medium spaghetti squash, about five cups cooked
- salt & fresh pepper for taste
- 1/3 cup of part-skim ricotta cheese
- 2 tbsp of grated parmesan cheese
- 1 tbsp of chopped parsley, or basil
- 3/4 cup of whole milk shredded mozzarella cheese

For the sauce:

- 1 tsp of olive oil
- A half finely chopped onion
- 3 cloves of minced garlic

- 14 oz of Italian chicken sausage
- 14 oz of a half can of crushed tomatoes (preferably Tuttorosso)
- Salt & fresh pepper, to taste
- Two tbsps. of chopped basil
- One bay of leaf

Directions

1. Preheat the furnace to 4000F.
2. Cut spaghetti squash in half & proceed to scoop out the seeds & membrane lengthwise. Lightly season with salt and black pepper; bake on a baking sheet for about 1 hour, or longer if necessary, cut side down.
3. Cut the squash in half size if you prefer the microwave, scoop out seeds and fibers, and place on

a safe microwave dish and cover. Microwave for eight to nine minutes or until soft.

4. Combine the ricotta cheese, 2 tablespoons of parmesan cheese, and parsley in a small bowl.
5. Heat the oil and add the onions and garlic in a large deep-frying pan; sauté on a medium-low for about 3 to 4 minutes, until soft.
6. Add the sausage and cook until browned and cooked through, breaking into smaller pieces.
7. Add the crushed tomatoes when cooked, and adjust the salt and pepper to taste. Add the bay leaf and the cover and reduce the heat to a low level.
8. Simmer for 20 to 30 minutes, then, at the very end, add fresh basil.
9. When cooking spaghetti squash, keep the oven on for about 10 minutes to keep it cool. Preheat the oven to 400 ° F if you've microwaved it.

10. Use a fork to remove flesh when the spaghetti squash is cool enough to handle, which will emerge out in spaghetti going to look strands reserving the shells.
11. To soak up any excess liquid, drain the squash on a paper towel, then toss it with half of the sauce. Return the spaghetti squash to the 6 shells and put it on a baking sheet.
12. Top each with the remaining sauce, 1 tablespoon of ricotta cheese mixture, and 2 tablespoons of mozzarella cheese. Bake in the oven for up till 30 mins or until the cheese is melted and everything is hot.

Asian Quinoa Meatballs

Preparation Time: 15 Minutes

Cook Time: 20 Minutes

Total Time: 35 Minutes

Yield: 20 Meatballs

Recipes:

- 1 pound of ground turkey
- 3/4 cup of cooked quinoa
- 3 cloves of garlic, minced
- Two green onions, thinly sliced
- One big egg
- One tablespoon of soy sauce
- Two teaspoons of sesame oil
- 1 teaspoon of Sriracha, or more, to taste
- Kosher salt & freshly ground black pepper for taste
- A half teaspoon of sesame seeds

For the sauce:

- A quarter cup of soy sauce
- Two tablespoons of rice vinegar
- 1 tablespoon of freshly grated ginger
- 1 tablespoon of brown sugar, packed
- 1 teaspoon of sesame oil
- 1 teaspoon of Sriracha, or more, to taste
- 2 teaspoons of cornstarch

Directions

1. Preheat the oven to 400°F. Lightly oil a 9/13 clean baking dish with nonstick spray or coat.
2. Combine onions, ground turkey, quinoa, garlic, egg, soy sauce, sesame oil, Sriracha, salt, and pepper in a large bowl, to taste.
3. Stir until well combined, using a clean wooden spoon or with clean hands. Roll 1 1/4-to-1 1/2-inch

meatballs into the mixture, forming about 18-20 meatballs.

4. Place meatballs on the prepared baking dish and bake for 18-20 minutes, or until browned and cooked through on all sides.
5. To make the sauce, whisk altogether soy sauce, sesame oil, rice vinegar, ginger, sugar, Sriracha & a half cup of water in a small saucepan over a medium-high heat.
6. Whisk the cornstarch and 1 tablespoon of water together in a small bowl. Stir until thickened, about 2 minutes into the soy sauce mixture.
7. Serve the meatballs, garnished with green onion and sesame seeds, with sauce immediately.

Herbed Turkey Burgers With Zucchini Buns

Preparation Time: 10 Minutes

Cook Time: 15 minutes

Total Time: 25 minutes

Yields: 2 Servings

Calories: 177kcal

Recipes:

- 8 to 10 oz of ground organic lean turkey meat
- 2 tablespoons of fresh oregano chopped
- Two minced garlic cloves
- 4 thick slices of zucchini
- Olive oil spray
- Salt & pepper to taste

Directions

1. Combine the turkey meat, oregano & garlic cloves in a large bowl, and mix until fully combined with your hands. Form and set aside into two patties.
2. Heat a medium-high heat grill pan (or outdoor grill).
3. Spray both sides with the zucchini and sprinkle with salt and pepper.
4. Add the zucchini to the grill pan, cook until you have nice grill marks, and the zucchini still retains its shape, 2-3 minutes per side.
5. Add the whole turkey burgers to the grill & cook until cooked, 3-5 minutes per side.
6. Serve between slices of zucchini and add your toppings of choice.
7. Serve to Enjoy!

Avocado Toast With Sunny Side Egg

Preparation TIME: 5 Minutes

COOK TIME: 5 Minutes

TOTAL TIME: 10 Minutes

Recipes:

- One slice of toasted whole-grain bread(1.5 oz)
- 1 oz of mashed, 1/4 small Haas avocado
- cooking spray
- 1 big egg
- kosher salt & black pepper to taste
- Hot sauce (optional)

Directions

1. In a small clean bowl, mash the avocado & season with salt and pepper.

2. Over low heat, heat a small nonstick skillet, spray it with oil, and gently crack the egg in the skillet. Cover and cook according to your taste.
3. Place the mashed avocado over the toast and, if desired, top with the egg, salt and pepper, and hot sauce!

30 Minute One Pan Chicken Fajitas

Preparation Time: 5 minutes

Cook Time: 15 minutes

Course: Main Course

Yields: 3 Servings

Calories: 215

Recipes:

- Two fresh bell peppers (cut into thin stripes)
- One-pound of boneless skinless chicken breasts or thighs cut into thin stripes.
- One teaspoon of chilli powder
- One onion (cut into thin stripes)
- Half teaspoon of black pepper
- One teaspoon of paprika

- One tablespoon of olive oil for cooking
- One teaspoon of ground cumin
- Half teaspoon of garlic salt

Directions

1. Firstly, you should mix chicken with spices in the clean medium container and set for fifteen minutes.
2. Now heat up oil in the large clean skillet over medium to high heat. Add vegetables to the skillet and then cook for around seven minutes, occasionally stirring.
3. Add chicken to the skillet and cook for an additional five to seven minutes until it is not pink anymore.
4. Serve with tortillas, over rice or with lettuce.

Buffalo Wing Turkey Lettuce Wraps

Preparation Time: 10 Minutes

Cook Time: 20 Minutes

Total Time: 30 Minutes

Recipes:

- Half cup of onion (diced finely)
- One-pound lean ground turkey
- 3/4 cup of carrot shavings (shavings can be done using a vegetable peeler)
- One teaspoon of minced garlic
- One head iceberg lettuce (leaves removed to form cups)
- One cup of celery (sliced thinly)

- Blue cheese crumbles or dressing to drizzle over the top (I used some one tablespoon of Litehouse Bleu Cheese Vinaigrette and blue cheese crumbles)
- Salt
- Half cup of Frank's Red Hot Buffalo wing sauce
- Pepper

Directions

1. Sauté the onions over medium heat in a large clean skillet until it gets soft (three to four mins). Add garlic and then cook for one additional minute. Add brown meat, ground turkey, season with pepper and salt, and cook until it is well cooked. Drain any grease if required.
2. Transfer meat back to pan and then stir in the wing sauce. Decrease the heat to low and then simmer for few minutes.

To Prepare lettuce:

1. Into lettuce cup, add a spoonful of meat, top with chopped celery and carrot shavings. Sprinkle with blue cheese crumbles with/ dressing. Wrap up and serve to eat!

Skinny Orange Chicken

Preparation Time: 10 Minutes

Cook Time: 10 Minutes

Total Time: 20 Minutes

Yields: 4 to 6 Servings

Recipes:

For Orange Chicken:

- Two tablespoons of olive oil
- Two-pounds boneless, skinless chicken breasts (cut into bite-sized pieces)
- Salt
- Pepper

Toppings:

- Toasted sesame seeds
- Orange zest
- Thinly sliced green onions

For Orange Chicken Sauce:

- Half cup of orange juice
- Three cloves garlic (minced)
- Half cup of honey
- 1/4 cup of rice wine vinegar
- 1/3 cup of soy sauce
- Half teaspoon of ground ginger
- Three tablespoon of cornstarch
- Half teaspoon of white pepper
- Pinch of crushed red pepper flakes
- Zest of one orange

Directions

To Make The Orange Chicken:

1. Chicken should be generously seasoned with pepper and salt.
2. Now heat up oil in a clean large saute pan over medium to high heat. Add chicken and saute for around four to six minutes, occasionally stirring, until the chicken appears browned and almost cooked through.
3. Pour in the orange chicken sauce, and stir to combine. Allow the sauce to boil, then boil for an additional one-minute or two until it gets thickened. Take away from the heat and serve straight away over rice. Garnish with sesame seeds, additional orange zest and green onions.

To Make The Orange Chicken Sauce:

Whisk all recipes together until thoroughly combined. For sauce to be way sweeter, simply add an extra two to four tablespoons of honey.

Grilled Chicken Sandwich With Avocado And Tomato

Course: Lunch

Calories: 253

Total Time: 15 Minutes

Yield: 1 Serving

Recipes:

- Two tablespoons of mashed avocado
- Two ounces Ciabatta
- Three slices of ripe tomatoes
- Fresh pepper as desired
- Two ounces grilled chicken breast
- Salt

Directions

1. Firstly slice bread open with a clean knife and smear mashed avocado on the bread. Season with salt and pepper.
2. Top with chicken, add additional fresh cracked pepper and tomatoes. Serve to enjoy!!

Avocado Kale Smoothie

Yields: 2 Servings

Recipes:

- Two cups of baby kale leaves
- 1 1/4 cup of coconut water
- Half cup of avocado
- Two teaspoons of fresh-squeezed lime juice
- One banana (frozen)

Directions

Firstly you should pour coconut water into a clean blender. Add avocado, kale, lime juice and frozen banana. Cover with lid and then blend until it is smooth. Pour into two clean glasses and serve straightaway.

Garlic Kale Chips

Recipes:

- One tablespoon of olive oil
- One bunch of fresh kale
- ¼ teaspoon of fresh ground pepper
- A pinch of cayenne pepper
- ¼ teaspoon of garlic powder
- ¼ teaspoon of salt

Directions

1. Firstly, heat up the oven to 300 degrees Fahrenheit and carefully line one to two large baking sheets with a clean parchment paper and put aside.
2. Gently rinse kale and then pat dry with clean paper towels. Afterwards, remove the thick stems and tear the leaves into bite-sized pieces.

3. In a large clean container combine salt, olive oil, garlic powder, cayenne pepper and pepper.

Kale, Broccoli, and Feta Sauté

Preparation Time: 25 Minutes

Total Time: 25 Minutes

Yields: 4 Servings

Recipes:

- Four cups of broccoli florets
- Three tablespoons of olive oil
- Black pepper
- Kosher salt
- ¼ cup of kalamata olives,(pitted and slivered)
- Two ounces (half cup) Feta (crumbled)
- One medium bunch (around ten cups) kale (thick stems removed and leaves torn into bite-size pieces)

Directions

1. Firstly, you should heat up the oil in a large clean skillet over medium to high heat. Add the broccoli, season with ¼ teaspoon of pepper and half teaspoon of salt, and then cook, occasionally tossing, until it gets tender, eight to ten minutes.
2. Now add the kale and then cook again, occasionally tossing until it gets tender, six to eight minutes extra. Fold in the Feta & olives.

Kale, Sesame and Ginger Salad

Preparation Time: 5 Minutes

Cook Time: 5 Minutes

Total Time: 10 Minutes

Yields: 4 Servings

Recipes:

- Two tablespoons of toasted sesame seeds
- One bunch of kale, washed and chopped into 2-inch pieces (ribs left on)
- Two tablespoons of toasted sesame oil
- 1/8 teaspoon of sea salt
- Two tablespoons of ginger (minced)
- 1/8 teaspoon of fresh ground pepper
- Two tablespoons of apple cider vinegar (raw preferably)

Directions

1. In a large clean container, prepare an ice bath (around twelve ice cubes and cold water). Put aside.
2. Boil four cups of water in a clean medium pot.
3. Blanche the kale in hot water, using tongs (for around thirty seconds) and instantly place into the cold, ice bath to s the cooking process. The leaves should appear bright green. Put aside to let it cool.
4. Make dressing in a small clean container by whisking the sesame oil, minced ginger, salt and apple cider vinegar.
5. Strain the kale to drain water. Toss with dressing and toasted sesame seeds.

5 Minute Vegan Kale Pesto

Preparation Time: 3 Minutes

Cook Time: 2 Minutes

Yields: (Two tablespoons each) 8 Servings

Recipes:

- Half cup of olive oil
- Two cups of torn kale (stems removed) and parsley, combined
- Half cup of raw almonds
- One clove garlic
- 1/4 teaspoon of salt (more as preferred)
- One lemon juice

Directions

1. Firstly, pulse the olive oil, kale, garlic, lemon juice and salt in a clean food processor until it gets smooth.
2. Add in almonds and then pulse again until the almonds are ground as preferred.
3. Serve with pasta, pizza, eggs, sandwiches, crackers, soup, salads, etc.

Skinny Buffalo Cauliflower Bites

Course: Appetizer

Preparation Time: 5 Minutes

Cook Time: 30 Minutes

Total Time: 35 Minutes

Yields: 4 to 6 Servings

Recipes:

- 3/4 cup of Frank's Red Hot Sauce
- One head Cauliflower (stems removed and chopped into bite size florets)
- One tablespoon of Honey
- One teaspoon of Garlic Powder
- 1/4 teaspoon of ground Black Pepper
- 1/4 teaspoon of ground Sea Salt

Directions

1. Firstly, heat up the oven to 450 degrees Fahrenheit.
2. In small clean container add Garlic Powder, Frank's Red Hot Sauce, Salt, Pepper and Honey. Stir to combine thoroughly.
3. In large clean ziplock bag, add Cauliflower florets and then pour sauce over Cauliflower.
4. Afterwards, seal bag and then move the Cauliflower around to make it coated with the sauce.
5. Add Cauliflower to a clean sheet pan carefully lined with a clean parchment paper or spray the clean pan with nonstick cooking spray instead of parchment paper. Bake for twenty to thirty minutes or determined by the florets you want.
6. Serve with Blue Cheese Dressing or Ranch.
7. Serve to enjoy!

Healthy Cauliflower Mashed Potatoes

Course: Side Dish

Preparation Time: 10 Minutes

Cook Time: 10 Minutes

Total Time: 20 Minutes

Yields: 4 Servings

Recipes:

- Three cloves garlic
- One medium head cauliflower (Three pounds) trimmed and cut into florets
- 1/8 teaspoon of ground black pepper (freshly)
- Half teaspoon of salt
- One tablespoon of extra virgin olive oil

For Garnish:

Extra virgin olive oil, Chopped fresh thyme, Freshly ground black pepper and Homemade flavored salt

Directions

1. Firstly, bring a large clean pot of salted water to a boil, add the garlic and cauliflower and then cook for around ten minutes or until it is the cauliflower is fork gets tender. Now drain, take back to the hot pan and with the lid on, let it stand for two to three minutes.
2. Move garlic and the cauliflower to a clean food processor, add the salt, pepper and olive oil and purée until it is smooth. (using a hand blender and potato masher is allowed).
3. salt and pepper just as desired.

4. Garnish with a drizzle of olive oil, salt, chopped fresh thyme and pepper.
5. Serve straightaway.

Note

The cauliflower-mashed potatoes can be stored in the refrigerator for up to three days.

Baked Brussels Sprouts Chips

Preparation Time: 10 Minutes

Cook Time: 5 Minutes

Total time: 15 Minutes

Yields: 4 Servings

Recipes:

- Sea salt (as desired)
- Two teaspoons of olive oil
- One pound Brussels sprouts

Directions

1. Firstly, you should heat up the oven to 350 degrees Fahrenheit.
2. Cut the bottom of a Brussels sprout off, using a small knife, so that a few of the outer leaves fall off.

Place the separated leaves into a medium clean container. Do it again until all the Brussels sprouts have been cut & leaves have been removed.

3. You peel all the Brussels sprouts immediately, toss the leaves with a small drizzle of olive oil and sea salt, and carefully layer them on a clean baking sheet in a single layer.
4. Lastly, bake the Brussels sprout leaves for around four to six minutes or until the tips begin appears lightly browned and the leaves are also crispy. Pay enough attention to avoid burning!

Shaved Brussels Sprout Salad with Apples & Walnuts

Preparation Time: 20 Minutes

Total Time: 20 Minutes

Yields: 6 Servings

Recipes:

For the Salad:

- One medium tart apple (like Granny Smith)
- One pound Brussels sprouts
- One cup of chopped walnuts
- One medium red onion

For the Vinaigrette:

- One tablespoon of Dijon mustard
- Two teaspoons of maple syrup
- Salt and pepper, as desired
- One clove garlic, finely minced
- Three tablespoons of red wine vinegar
- Half cup of extra virgin olive oil

Directions

1. Firstly, you should trim the ends off the Brussels sprouts. Slice each sprout thinly with a shape knife. Also slice the red onion and apple in the same way. Combine in a large clean container.
2. Now, toast the walnuts in a clean skillet over medium to high heat, frequently stirring, until it begins to fragrant and also appears lightly browned,

around two minutes. To the mixture, add brussels sprouts. Toss to combine well.

3. Combine the vinaigrette recipes into a clean jar with a tigh lid. Carefully close the lid and then shake until it is well combined.
4. Afterwards, pour over the Brussels sprout mixture, and toss to make it coat. Place in the refrigerator for around thirty minutes before serving it.

Roasted Brussels Sprouts And Cauliflower Soup

Course: Soup, Lunch, Dinner

Calories: 173

Preparation Time: 5 Minutes

Cook Time: 30 Minutes

Total Time: 35 Minutes

Yields: 4 Servings

Recipes:

- 16 ounces cauliflower florets
- Canola cooking spray
- 16 ounces brussels sprouts, halved
- Black pepper (as desired)
- One teaspoon of butter, or more oil for DF, W30,

- Two tablespoons of olive oil
- Half cup of chopped shallots
- 3/4 teaspoon of kosher salt
- 3 1/2 cups of vegetable broth

Directions

1. Firstly, heat up the oven to 450 degrees Fahrenheit.
2. Carefully line a large baking sheet with a clean foil and also spray with oil. Place the Brussels and cauliflower cut side down on the clean baking sheet, drizzle with oil and then roast on the bottom third of the oven twenty-five minutes, tossing halfway until it appears slightly browned.
3. Proceed to melt the butter in a big clean saucepan over low heat and then add shallots. Cook until it appears translucent, around five minutes. Add the

broth and the salt and then simmer for another five minutes.

4. Put off the oven, keep around one cup of the roasted vegetables and store it warm on the baking sheet.
5. Move the rest to the pot and then simmer for additional two minutes.
6. Transfer in 2 groups to a clean blender and then blend until it gets smooth.
7. Serve in four containers topped with fresh black pepper and the roasted vegetables as desired. Serve straight away.

Butternut Squash Coleslaw with Honey Goat Cheese Dressing

Preparation Time: 15 Minutes

Total Time: 15 Minutes

Yields: 4 Servings

Recipes:

- One and a half tablespoons honey
- 4 oz. fresh creamy goat cheese, room temperature
- Two teaspoons of apple cider vinegar
- Three tablespoons of extra-virgin olive oil
- Kosher salt
- Half lemon juice
- Freshly ground black pepper
- Half cup of toasted walnuts

- One medium butternut squash
- Two tablespoons of chopped parsley leaves
- Half cup of dried cranberries

Required Equipment:

- Mandoline

Directions

1. Combine honey, goat cheese, vinegar, olive oil, and lemon juice; in a large clean mixing container, and then season with some salt and enough freshly ground black pepper. Stir with a whisk until it is totally combined and also creamy.
2. Get rid of the top narrow part of the butternut squash and then peel. Using a sharp knife or a mandoline , cut the peeled cylinder into fine long matchsticks (should make around four cups). Fold

into the cheese dressing along with walnuts, chopped fresh parsley and dried cranberries.

Butternut Squash Hash Browns

Course: Breakfast

Recipes:

- Half onion finely chopped
- One butternut squash, peeled (shredded using food processor)
- One tablespoon of coconut oil
- Five to Six strips pork or turkey bacon
- Half teaspoon of garlic powder or more to taste
- One tablespoon of maple syrup
- Five to Six drops fresh lemon juice
- Half to One teaspoon of sea salt or more, to taste

Directions

1. Heat the oil in a clean frying pan and then add bacon to fry until it is well cooked (four minutes, or

thereabout, for each side) and remove to a single dish. Leave the bacon grease in the pan.

2. Add onion to pan and then cook for five minutes until it gets tender.
3. Add squash to pan, the spices and then sauté for twenty minutes or so, until it is done. Add maple syrup and stir to combine. Taste, add five drops of lemon juice. Taste once more.
4. Add extra salt, lemon and syrup.
5. Top with crumble bacon and enjoy.

Parmesan Butternut Squash Fries

Preparation Time: 15 Minutes

Cook Time: 30 Minutes

Total Time: 45 Minutes

Yields: 6 Servings

Recipes:

- One tablespoon of olive oil
- One medium butternut squash, peeled, seeded and cut into half-inch thick matchsticks
- Half teaspoon of dried oregano
- 1/4 cup of freshly grated Parmesan cheese
- Half teaspoon of dried thyme
- Kosher salt
- A pinch of cayenne pepper
- Two tablespoons of chopped fresh chives

- Freshly ground black pepper, to taste

Directions:

1. Firstly, you should heat up oven to 425 degrees Fahrenheit. Coat a cooling rack with clean nonstick spray and place on a clean baking sheet; put aside.
2. Gently place the butternut squash in a single layer onto the readied baking sheet. Add thyme, olive oil, cayenne pepper and oregano; season with pepper and salt, to desired. Carefully toss to combine.
3. Now place into the oven and then bake for twenty-five to thirty minutes, or until it appears golden brown and also crispy.
4. Garnish with chives and top with Parmesan, if wanted. Serve straightaway.

Roasted Butternut Squash Hummus

Preparation Time: 10 Minutes

Cook Time: 30 Minutes

Total Time: 40 Minutes

Yields: 8 Servings

Recipes:

- Two tablespoons of olive oil
- One and a half cups of roasted butternut squash (instructions for roasting below)
- Two tablespoons of tahini
- One and a half cups cooked chickpeas (rinsed and drained)
- One lemon juice
- One garlic clove, peeled
- Two tablespoons of water

- Half teaspoon of sea salt
- 1/4 teaspoon of smoked paprika
- Freshly ground pepper
- 1/4 teaspoon of cumin

Directions

1. Firstly, you should heat up the oven to 425 degrees Fahrenheit.
2. Butternut squash cut into halves and then scoop out seeds
3. Rub one teaspoon of olive oil over insides of butternut squash (half teaspoon on each halves).
4. Place the olive oil-rubbed-side down on a clean baking sheet and then roast for about thirty minutes.
5. Bring out from the oven & allow it to cool.

6. As soon as it is cooled, scoop out one and a half cups.
7. Add chickpeas, one and a half tablespoon of olive oil, butternut squash, garlic, tahini, water and lemon to blender or a clean food processor and process until it gets smooth.
8. Add in spices and continue blending until it is well combined.
9. Serve with crackers (or dipping of choice) and veggies.

Note:

It can be preserved in refrigerator for about one week.

Squash leftovers can be scooped out and stored in the refrigerator.

Beet & Berry Smoothie

Course: Smoothie

Preparation Time: 10 Minutes

Total Time: 10 Minutes

Yields: 4 Servings

Recipes:

- One frozen banana
- One cup of plant milk of choice or water
- One cup of frozen or fresh strawberries
- One tablespoon of hemp seeds (if desired)
- One small beet, washed, peeled, and cut into sixths
- One cup of frozen or fresh blueberries

Directions

Add all recipes to a clean blender, and blend for two to three minutes or until it gets smooth. Pulse is recommended on your blender if it can. Then, blend steadily until it smoothens.

Beet Slaw

Preparation Time: 20 Minutes

Total Time: 25 Minutes

Recipes:

- 1/3 cup of scallion stalks (thinly sliced)
- Three to Four large raw beets (peeled and grated)
- 1/4 cup of mint (finely chopped)
- One-inch chunk ginger (peeled and grated)
- One tablespoon of honey (For vegan sub maple syrup for honey)
- Half lemon juiced
- 1/3 cup of golden raisins
- One tablespoon of apple cider vinegar
- 1/3 cup of sliced raw almonds
- One tablespoon of sesame seeds (if desired)

- One pinch of fine sea salt

Directions

1. Firstly, grate ginger and beets.
2. In a large clean container toss all recipes together and mix to combine well.
3. Serve straight away or store in an airtight container in the refrigerator for six hours until before serving.

Olive Oil-Baked Beet Chips With Sea Salt & Black Pepper

Yields: 2 to 4 Servings

Recipes:

- Two tablespoons of olive oil
- Two pounds large beets (peeled)
- Freshly cracked black pepper
- Sea salt

Directions

1. Firstly, you should heat up the oven to 350 Fahrenheit. Gently line several baking sheets with clean parchment paper.
2. Slice beets thinly to a thickness of 1/16-inches, using a mandoline. In a large clean container, toss beet slices with oil to coat equally.

3. On arranged baking sheets, in a single layer, place enough slices as will fit. Bake until it is crispy, twenty-five to thirty minutes, rotating pans once between while baking. Cool chips and blot with clean paper towels to eliminate any surplus oil. Do it again, using a cool readied baking sheet for every batch, until all the beet slices are also baked.
4. Toss the chips with 1/4 teaspoon of pepper and salt or just as desired.

Beet, Ginger, and Coconut Milk Soup

Yields: 4 Servings

Recipes:

- One large yellow onion, diced
- One tablespoon of olive oil
- One tablespoon of finely chopped ginger
- Three cloves garlic, finely chopped
- Five cups of vegetable stock, divided
- Three large red beets, peeled and cut into 1/4-inch pieces
- Half teaspoon of fine sea salt
- One can (14.5 ounces) low-fat coconut milk
- Crusty bread (if desired)
- Parsley (if desired)
- 1/4 teaspoon of ground black pepper (freshly)

- Canned julienned beets (if desired)

Directions

1. In a large clean pot; heat up oil over medium heat. Sauté onion, for about five minutes. Add ginger and garlic; cook, often stirring, five minutes.
2. Add four cups of stock and beets; bring to a boil, then decrease heat and then simmer until it is beets are fork-tender, twenty minutes.
3. With regular blender and an immersion, puree soup, adding remaining one cup of stock as required to reach preferred taste.
4. Stir in salt, pepper and milk. Garnish with parsley and julienned beets and serve with bread, if desired.

Cilantro Pesto over Zucchini Noodles

Preparation Time: 15 Minutes

Total Time: 15 Minutes

Yield: 2 Cups

Recipes:

- Half cup of cashews (lightly roasted)
- Two bunches (four-ounces) of cilantro (Coarsely chop, leaving enough of the stems behind)
- Two tablespoons of olive oil or maybe avocado oil
- Two avocados (peeled and pitted)
- Four cloves of garlic minced
- Two teaspoons of sea salt
- About three cups of freshly chopped tomatoes
- One recipe of Zucchini Noodles

Directions

1. On a low speed in a clean blender, combine all the recipes and then blend using the tamper to maintain the mixture moving. Should take some minutes before the pesto turned out to be justly smooth.
2. If you're using a food processor: process all ingredients, scraping down the sides as necessary until the pesto is mostly smooth.
3. Serve straight away as preferred or with freshly chopped tomatoes and a recipe of Zucchini Noodles.

Mexican Cauliflower (Rice)

Course: Side Dish

Calories: 58

Preparation Time: 5 Minutes

Cook Time: 5 Minutes

Total Time: 10 Minutes

Yield: 4 Servings

Recipes:

- One teaspoon of olive oil
- Four cups of cauliflower crumbles (purchase at any store)
- Two medium plum tomatoes (small dice)
- Half medium onion (finely diced)
- Two garlic cloves (minced)

- One jalapeno (seeds & membrane removed, minced)
- Half teaspoon of cumin
- Two tablespoons of tomato paste
- Chopped cilantro
- ¼ teaspoon of cayenne pepper
- One teaspoon of kosher salt
- ¼ teaspoon of smoked paprika
- Freshly ground black pepper (as desired)

Directions

1. Firstly, you should heat up the oil in a large clean skillet over medium to high heat. Once it is hot, add tomatoes, jalapeno and the onions and sauté until it gets just tender, around two to three minutes. Add the cauliflower and garlic, sauté until the cauliflower becomes just tender, two minutes.

2. Add the cumin, tomato paste, cayenne, paprika, pepper and salt. Stir to equally coat the vegetables and cook for one minute or until it is heated through. Top with the chopped cilantro and then serve to enjoy.

Thai Red Curry Cauliflower Rice

Preparation Time: 10 Minutes

Cook Time: 15 Minutes

Total Time: 25 Minutes

Yield: 4 Servings

Recipes:

- Half white onion (diced)
- Half teaspoon of coconut oil
- One tablespoon of fresh ginger (peeled and minced)
- Three cloves garlic (minced)
- Five small carrots (peeled and diced)
- One jalapeño (minced)
- One red bell pepper (diced)
- Two tablespoons of Thai Kitchen Red Curry Paste

- One cup of green peas
- One head of cauliflower, riced
- Two tablespoons of soy sauce or tamari
- One cup Thai Kitchen Lite Coconut Milk (shake vigorously before opening)
- Pepper
- Salt

Directions

1. In clean pan, add coconut oil and then bring to medium heat. Add, ginger, garlic, jalapeño, carrot and onion.
2. Sauté, often stirring, for around five minutes until it starts to gets soften.
3. Add red curry paste, cauliflower and red pepper and stir to combine.

4. Add soy sauce and coconut milk and then stir to combine.
5. Cook for approximately ten minutes, frequently stirring, until they all get softened and the carrots also becoming tender.
6. Add in green peas then stir, let it cook for additional one or two minutes.
7. Serve straight away with fresh cilantro and chopped green onion.

Raw Rainbow "Noodles"

Yields: 4 Servings

Recipes:

- Two large maroon carrots
- Two large orange carrots
- One large sweet apple
- One medium parsnip
- Three scallions
- One piece of fresh ginger about 2-inches long
- One tablespoon of apple cider vinegar
- 1/4 cup of toasted pecans chopped
- One tablespoon of maple syrup
- Pepper
- Two tablespoons of olive oil
- Kosher salt

Directions

1. The vegetables and apple should be peeled and shredded using a mandoline or other available shredding tool.
2. Proceed to peel the ginger and shred around one tablespoon (or more or less to taste).
3. Slice the scallions into two-inch pieces, and then slice each piece in half the length.
4. Place all in a clean container, and toss with pecans to ensure it combines so well.
5. Mix syrup, vinegar, olive oil and then season with pepper and salt as preferred.
6. Proceed to pour the dressing over the salad and then toss to coat well.
7. You should refrigerate for around thirty minutes allow the flavours to develop, and then serve to enjoy.

Raw Carrot Pasta With Ginger-Lime Peanut Sauce

Course: Main Course

Calories: 111

Preparation Time: 15 Minutes

Total Time: 15 Minutes

Yields: 6 Servings

Recipes:

For The Carrot Pasta:

- 1/3 cup of roasted cashews
- Two tablespoons of fresh cilantro finely chopped
- Five large carrots (peeled and spiraled into noodles)

For The Ginger-Lime Peanut Sauce:

- Four tablespoons of coconut milk
- Two tablespoons of unsweetened creamy peanut butter or almond butter
- A pinch cayenne pepper
- Two tablespoons of liquid aminos
- Kosher salt (as desired)
- Two cloves large garlic finely chopped
- One tablespoon of lime juice
- One tablespoon of fresh ginger peeled and grated

Directions:

To Prepare The Ginger-Lime Peanut Sauce:

1. Combine all recipes in a small clean container and mix together until it is smooth and gets creamy.

To Prepare The Carrot Pasta:

1. Rinse and peel the carrots, and then pat dry afterwards.
2. Create noodles from the carrots, with a spiral slicer. You can grate the carrots when you have small inches left.
3. Move all carrot noodles into a large clean serving dish. Add the Ginger-Lime Peanut Sauce over the noodles and carefully toss to combine.
4. Serve with freshly chopped cilantro and roasted cashews (or peanuts).

Tahini Dill Carrot Noodles

Recipes:

- ¼ cup of tahini
- Eight to ten large carrots
- Two tablespoons of lemon juice
- One tablespoon of chopped dill
- One teaspoon of garlic powder
- Four tablespoons of water
- One teaspoon of lemon zest
- One teaspoon of salt

Directions

1. Continuously peel the carrots and get rid of the scraps.
2. In a large clean container, place the carrot ribbons and then put aside.

3. In a small clean container combine dill, tahini, water, lemon juice, salt and garlic powder. Add the water depending on how thick you want the tahini to be.
4. Pour around half of the sauce over the noodles and toss to combine thoroughly. Add extra if you prefer it thicker.
5. Now garnish with lemon zest and then serve to enjoy.

Raw Beet and Sweet Potato Salad

Preparation Time: 10 Minutes

Total Time: 10 Minutes

Yields: 6 Servings

Recipes:

- One-bunch beets (Three to Four)
- Garlic Lime Vinaigrette
- Two large sweet potatoes
- Half cup toasted pepitas pumpkins seeds
- Four scallions

Directions

1. Firstly, you should peel the beets and sweet potatoes. Now cut the veggies into long curly strips, using a spiralizer .

2. Proceed to cut the pieces into convenient lengths, with a pair of kitchen shears.
3. Mix the sweet potato ribbons and beets in a large clean container. Afterwards, cut the scallion tops at an angle to create long rings.
4. Lastly, sprinkle the salad with pepitas and scallions. Serve along with the desired vinaigrette.

One Pot Italian Eggplant Noodle Parmesan

Preparation Time: 25 Minutes

Cook Time: 20 Minutes

Total Time: 45 minutes

Yields: 6 Servings

Recipes:

- 25 cherry tomatoes (seeds removed and quartered)
- Two long eggplants (cut into thin long noodle size strips)
- One or two cloves of garlic (chopped)
- 1/4 cup plus two tablespoons of olive oil
- Eight small mozzarella balls chopped
- One pinch or two hot pepper flakes (optional)

- Half teaspoon of oregano
- 1/4 cup of freshly grated Parmesan cheese
- Four to five leaves fresh basil chopped

Directions

1. Add eggplant noodles and one teaspoon of salt in a large clean container and then toss, let it sit for around twenty to thirty minutes, and then rinse and drain it well. Make the sauce whilst eggplants are sitting.
2. In a large clean pan add garlic, 1/4 cup of oil, oregano, cherry tomatoes, a pinch of salt, hot pepper flakes and basil, cook on medium heat for roughly ten minutes (until tomatoes become soft and liquid also gets evaporated).
3. Add two tablespoons of oil and well-drained eggplant noodles, toss to combine, cover and then

cook for five minutes, take away the lid and then cook for roughly five minutes or until the noodles gets soft (but isn't mushy), add parmesan cheese and mozzarella, carefully toss. Serve straight away.

4. Top with more Parmesan cheese if wanted. Enjoy!

Turkey Taco Lettuce Wraps

Course: Lunch, Dinner

Calories: 255

Preparation Time: 10 Minutes

Cook Time: 35 Minutes

Total Time: 45 Minutes

Yield: 4 Servings

Recipes:

- One teaspoon of garlic powder
- 1.3 pounds ground turkey (99 percent lean)
- One teaspoon of salt
- One teaspoon of cumin
- One teaspoon of paprika
- One teaspoon of chili powder

- Half small onion, minced
- Half teaspoon of oregano
- 3/4 cup of water
- Two tablespoons of bell pepper, minced
- Half cup of shredded reduced fat cheddar (if desired, you should neglect for Whole30)
- Eight large lettuce leaves from Iceberg lettuce
- Four ounces of can tomato sauce

Directions

1. In a large clean skillet add brown turkey smashing it into smaller pieces. As soon as it isn't pink anymore add dry seasoning and then mix well to combine.
2. Add the pepper, onion, tomato sauce and water, and then cover. Now simmer on low heat for around twenty minutes.
3. Now rise and then dry the lettuce.

4. Lastly, you should split the meat evenly between the eight leaves and then place in the middle of each leaf and top with your desired taco fixings and enjoy!

Curried Cauliflower Steaks with Red Rice & Tzatziki

Calories: 504

Active Time: 30 minutes

Total Time: 1 hour

Yields: 4 Servings

Recipes:

- ¾ cup of nonfat plain Greek yogurt
- Tzatziki
- One tablespoon of lemon juice
- ¼ cup of sour cream
- Half teaspoon of kosher salt
- One clove garlic, minced
- Rice and Cauliflower Steaks

- Half medium cucumber, seeded and grated
- 1/3 cup of extra-virgin olive oil
- One cup red rice or brown basmati rice
- Two teaspoons of curry powder
- Two tablespoons chopped fresh cilantro
- One tablespoon of lemon juice
- Two medium heads cauliflower
- Half teaspoon of kosher salt

Directions

To Prepare Tzatziki:

1. Whisk sour cream, yogurt, garlic, salt and lemon juice in a medium clean container until it gets smooth. Now, fold in the cucumber and then place in the refrigerator.

To Prepare Rice and Cauliflower:

1. Firstly, you should heat up the oven to 450 degrees Fahrenheit. Now gently line a large rimmed baking sheet with clean foil.
2. Cook rice following to package instructions. Store warm.
3. Meanwhile, whisk lemon juice, oil, salt and curry powder in a small clean container.
4. Get rid of all outer leaves from the cauliflower, however, keep stems. Place with stem-side down on a clean chopping board. Cut 2 one-inch-thick slices from the middle of each to get four (steaks) cauliflowers, with a large clean knife.
5. Cut enough of the cauliflower left into 3/4-inch florets to make four cups. Place the cauliflowers (steaks) and florets in just a single layer on the

readied clean baking sheet. Then, you should brush all sides with the curry mixture.

6. Now roast, gently turning, until the florets appear to be lightly browned and also the (steak stems) cauliflower gets tender, thirty to thirty-five minutes.
7. Refrigerate six tablespoons of tzatziki and the florets for later.
8. Split the rice in four dishes and then top each dish with 1/4 cup of tzatziki, a sprinkle of cilantro and a cauliflower steak.

Note

To Prepare Ahead:

You can refrigerate tzatziki (the prepared tzatziki) for about five days and also refrigerate the roasted cauliflower florets for about three days.

Tips:

You can make "*Curried Cauliflower Salad*" for lunch from the leftovers.

Directions

1. Combine half teaspoon of curry powder, six tablespoons of leftover tzatziki and one sliced scallion.
2. Coarsely chop the kept roasted cauliflower florets; stir into the sauce with 1/4 cup of rinsed canned chickpeas and 1/3 cup of diced cucumber.
3. Garnished with a six-inch whole-wheat pita and cilantro and then serve to enjoy.

Spaghetti Squash with Roasted Tomatoes, Beans and Almond Pesto

Calories: 502

Active: 45 Minutes

Total: 45 Minutes

Yields: 4 Servings

Recipes:

- Two cups of fresh basil leaves
- Almond Pesto
- Half cup of grated Parmesan cheese
- One cup of fresh parsley leaves
- ¼ cup of water
- One clove garlic
- ⅓ cup of whole raw almonds

- ¼ teaspoon of kosher salt
- One and half tablespoons red-wine vinegar
- ¼ cup of extra-virgin olive oil
- ¼ teaspoon of ground pepper

For Spaghetti Squash and Vegetables:

- ¼ cup of water
- One (3-pound) spaghetti squash
- One tablespoon of extra-virgin olive oil
- Two pints grape tomatoes, halved
- ¼ teaspoon of kosher salt
- One cup of canned cannellini beans, rinsed
- ¼ teaspoon of ground pepper

Directions

To Prepare Pesto:

1. Pulse parsley, basil, almonds, Parmesan, vinegar, 1/4 teaspoon each salt, pepper and garlic in a clean food processor until it is coarsely chopped, scraping down all sides. With the motor still functioning, add 1/4 cup of oil; process until it is well-combined.
2. Add water to the pesto; pulse to combine.

To Prepare Squash and Vegetables:

1. Firstly, you should heat up the oven to 400 degrees Fahrenheit. Gently line a rimmed baking sheet with clean foil.
2. Halve squash end-to-end and then remove the seeds. in a microwave place cut-side down in a plate and then add some water. Microwave at high until

the flesh can be effortlessly scraped using a fork, around fifteen minutes.

3. Now toss tomatoes with salt, pepper and oil in a large clean container. Move to the readied baking sheet.
4. Continue roasting until it gets soft and also wrinkled, ten to twelve minutes. Take out from the oven.
5. Add beans and then stir to combine well.
6. Now scrape the squash flesh into the container and split into four dishes. Top each part with some of the around three tablespoons of pesto sauce and tomato-bean mixture.

Note

To Prepare Ahead:

Pesto can be kept in the refrigerator pesto for about five days.

Tips:

You can make "*Pesto-Turkey Sandwich*" for lunch from the leftovers

Directions:

1. Spread one and a half tablespoon of leftover pesto on two slices toasted whole-wheat bread.
2. Top with two tomato slices, two lettuce leaves and three ounces of sliced deli turkey.

Salmon with Roasted Red Pepper Quinoa Salad

Calories: 481

Active: 15 Minutes

Total: 15 Minutes

Yields: 4 Servings

Recipes:

- 1-¼ pounds of skin-on salmon (preferably wild and cut into 4 portions)
- Three tablespoons of extra-virgin olive oil (divided)
- Half teaspoon of ground pepper (divided)
- Half teaspoon of salt (divided)
- One clove garlic (grated)
- Two tablespoons of red-wine vinegar

- ¼ cup of chopped fresh cilantro
- Two cups of cooked quinoa (directions below)
- ¼ cup of chopped toasted pistachios
- One cup of chopped roasted red bell peppers (from a twelve-ounce jar), washed

Directions

1. Firstly you should heat up one tablespoon of oil in a clean cast-iron skillet or large clean nonstick over medium to high heat. Gently pat salmon dry and then sprinkle the flesh with 1/4 teaspoon of both pepper and salt. Add skin-side up to the pan, and then cook until it gets lightly browned, three to four minutes. Turn and then cook until it's fairly cooked and flakes easily with a fork, one to two minutes more. Move to a clean dish.

2. Now whisk the left 1/4 teaspoon of both pepper and salt, two tablespoons of oil, vinegar and garlic in a medium clean container. Add peppers, quinoa, pistachios and cilantro; toss to combine. Serve the salmon with the salad.

Note

Store a pack of frozen cooked quinoa to add whole grains to dinner in a flash. Shelf-stable packets are excellent choice, too, but too rich in sodium, so it's a worry for you.

Loaded Spinach Salad

Calories: 484

Total Time: 40 Minutes

Yields: 2 Servings

Recipes:

For The Creamy Blue Cheese Dressing:

- ⅓ cup of low-fat mayonnaise
- ⅓ cup of buttermilk or nonfat milk
- ⅓ cup of nonfat plain yogurt
- Two tablespoons tarragon vinegar or white vinegar
- One tablespoon of Dijon mustard
- Half teaspoon of salt
- Half teaspoon of freshly ground pepper
- ¼ cup of crumbled blue cheese

For The Salad:

- Eight large eggs
- Six cups of baby spinach
- Four tablespoons Creamy Blue Cheese Dressing, divided
- 1 ounce 1 8-ounce can beets, rinsed and sliced
- One cup of shredded carrots
- 2 tablespoons 2 tablespoons chopped pecans, toasted (see notes below)

Directions

To Prepare Dressing:

1. Whisk buttermilk (or milk), mayonnaise, vinegar, yogurt, salt, pepper and mustard, in a medium clean container until it gets smooth. Add cheese and then

stir, mash using a spoon until the cheese is well combined.

To Prepare Salad:

1. In a clean saucepan, place eggs in a single layer; cover with enough water. And then bring to simmer over medium to high heat. Decrease the heat to low, cover and then cook at the lowermost simmer for ten minutes. Discard the hot water and then run cold water over the eggs until they are entirely cooled.
2. Discard six of the yolks after to peeling the eggs; Chop the remaining whites and yolks.
3. Toss two tablespoons of the dressing and spinach in a large clean container. Split between two plates.
4. Top with the beets, chopped eggs, pecans and carrots. Sprinkle with two additional tablespoons of

the dressing. (Store the extra dressing in the refrigerator for up to one week.)

Note

To Prepare Ahead:

1 1/4 cups of dressing are made from the recipes; cover and then refrigerate surplus dressing for about one week. Stir before making use of it again.

Tip:

To Toast Chopped Nuts:

You should cook in a small dry clean skillet over medium to low heat, constantly stirring, until it begins to fragrant and also appears lightly browned, two to four minutes.

Sheet-Pan Chicken Fajitas

Calories: 505

Active Time: 20 Minutes

Total Time: 40 Minutes

Yields: 4 Servings

Recipes:

- Two tablespoons of extra-virgin olive oil
- One-pound boneless, skinless chicken breasts
- One tablespoon of chili powder
- One teaspoon of garlic powder
- Two teaspoons of ground cumin
- One tablespoon of lime juice
- One large red bell pepper, sliced
- ¾ teaspoon of salt

- One large yellow bell pepper, sliced
- Eight corn tortillas (warmed)
- Two cups of sliced red or yellow onion (about 1 large)

For Serving:

- Sour cream
- Avocado and/or Pico de Gallo
- Cilantro
- Lime wedges

Directions

1. Firstly, you should heat up the oven to 400 degrees Fahrenheit. Using a cooking spray, gently coat a large rimmed clean baking sheet.
2. Proceed to cut the chicken breasts into halves (horizontally), and then also slice crosswise into strips. Combine chili powder, oil, cumin, and salt and garlic powder in a large clean container.
3. Now add the chicken and then stir to coat well with the spice mixture. Add onion and bell peppers and then stir once again to combine.
4. Move the vegetables and chicken to the set baking sheet and then gently spread in an even layer.
5. Now you should roast in the centre rack for fifteen minutes. While the pan is still there, turn the broiler to high heat. Continue to broil until the chicken is well cooked and the vegetables are also browning in

spots, around five minutes more. Take out from the oven.

6. Stir in the lime juice.
7. Serve the vegetables and chicken in warmed tortillas complemented by the lime wedges and then topped with avocado and/or pico de gallo and cilantro if desired.

Curried Scallop-Apple Salad

Calories: 487

Total Time: 25 Minutes

Yields: 4 Servings

Recipes:

- Six teaspoons of extra-virgin olive oil, divided
- Half cup of thinly sliced shallot
- ¾ teaspoon of curry powder
- One cup of apple cider
- Half teaspoon of salt (divided)
- One teaspoon of cider vinegar
- One pound of dry sea scallops,, tough muscle removed
- ¼ teaspoon freshly ground pepper
- Eight cups of mixed salad greens

- One tart apple, such as Granny Smith, diced
- ¼ cup of dried cranberries
- ¼ cup 1/4 cup sliced almonds, toasted (see Tip)

Directions

1. Firstly, you should heat up two teaspoons of oil in a large clean nonstick skillet over medium heat. Add curry powder and shallot and then cook, occasionally stirring, until the shallot is starting to soften, around three minutes. Add 1/4 teaspoon of salt and cider. Bring to a boil and then cook until decreased to 3/4 cup, around four minutes.
2. Pour into a large clean container and whisk in vinegar and two teaspoons of oil. Store 1/4 cup of the dressing in a small clean container. Then wipe out the pan when you are done.

3. Now you should pat scallops dry and then sprinkle with the left ¼ teaspoon of pepper and salt. Add the left two teaspoons of oil to the pan and heat over medium to high. Add the scallops and then cook until it appears golden brown, two to three minutes for each side. Move to a clean plate.
4. Add apple, salad greens, almonds and cranberries to the large container; then toss to coat well.
5. Top with the scallops and then drizzle with the store 1/4 cup of dressing.

Note

Tip:

You should carefully place sliced almonds in a small dry clean skillet and then cook over medium to low heat, constantly stirring, until it begins to fragrant and also appears lightly browned, two to four minutes.

Taco Lettuce Wraps

Calories: 510

Total Time: 30 Minutes

Yields: 4 Servings

Recipes:

- One tablespoon of canola oil
- Eight small iceberg or four large (cut in half crosswise) or romaine lettuce leaves
- ¼ teaspoon of salt
- One pound of lean ground beef
- One tablespoon of rice vinegar
- Five tablespoons of prepared salsa
- ¼ cup of finely diced red onion
- One cup of diced avocado
- 1 1/2 teaspoons of ground cumin

- A cup of julienned jícama (see note below)

Directions

1. Firstly you should wash and dry the lettuce leaves well and then cut out tough ribs.
2. Now you have to heat up oil in a large clean nonstick skillet over medium to high heat. Add ground beef and carefully season with salt and then cook, frequently stirring, until it is well cooked, four to six minutes.
3. Now whisk vinegar, cumin and salsa in a small clean container.
4. Take away the pan from the heat, and then add the salsa mixture and stir to combine well.
5. You can serve in the lettuce leaves, topped with jicama, onion and avocado.

Note

Jícama is a round root vegetable with fine brown skin and crunchy white flesh. The taste is mildly sweet and nutty. Use a small clean sharp knife or vegetable peeler to peel it, making sure to scrape both the papery brown skin and just below the fibrous flesh layer.

Conclusion

This Cookbook would serve as a guide to weight loss. The recipes are adequate for all cooking skill levels and are great to prepare with the families.

Lose weight and stay healthy.

Enjoy!

Printed in Great Britain
by Amazon

59323835R00145